Cardiac Arrhythmia Recognition
An easy learning guide

Easy Learning Guides from M&K

The array of complex functions carried out by senior clinical staff can be quite bewildering to more junior staff. Some of them would like to wave a magic wand that makes them instantly knowledgeable and confident. These *Easy Learning Guides* are not a magic wand, but they are probably the next best thing! They were written by a health professional who had to learn by experience, along with everyone else, but who knows that there are far easier ways to pick up these essential skills.

These no-fuss practical guides promote confidence and competence in several key areas of clinical practice, including:

Haemodynamic Monitoring and Manipulation

Arterial Blood Gas Analysis

Cardiac Arrhythmia Recognition

To find out more about these and other books published by M&K, as well as their wide range of clinical training courses, visit:
www.mkupdate.co.uk

Cardiac Arrhythmia Recognition

An easy learning guide

Fiona Foxall MA, RGN, ENB100, DPSN, BSc, PGCE

Lecturer in Nursing, Curtin University, Perth, Western Australia

With original artwork by Helen Blackburn

Cardiac Arrhythmia Recognition:
An Easy Learning Guide
Fiona Foxall

ISBN: 978-1-905539-53-6

First published 2010

British Library Catalogue in Publication Data
A catalogue record for this book is available from the British Library

Notice:
Clinical practice and medical knowledge constantly evolve. Standard safety precautions must be followed, but, as knowledge is broadened by research, changes in practice, treatment and drug therapy may become necessary or appropriate. Readers must check the most current product information provided by the manufacturer of each drug to be administered and verify the dosages and correct administration, as well as contraindications. It is the responsibility of the practitioner, utilising the experience and knowledge of the patient, to determine dosages and the best treatment for each individual patient. Any brands mentioned in this book are as examples only and are not endorsed by the Publisher. Neither the Publisher nor the author assume any liability for any injury and/or damage to persons or property arising from this publication.

The Publisher
To contact M&K Publishing write to:
M&K Update Ltd · The Old Bakery · St. John's Street
Keswick · Cumbria CA12 5AS
Tel: 01768 773030 · Fax: 01768 781099
publishing@mkupdate.co.uk
www.mkupdate.co.uk

Designed and typeset in Adobe Garamond 10/12 by S. Maria Hampshire.
Cover design by Luke Kelsey.

Printed in England by Reeds Printers, Penrith, Cumbria.

DEDICATION

For Mom and Dad.

Love always.

Contents

Acknowledgements

I would like to thank Mel Humphreys for her help with parts of this book and Maria Hampshire for her unfailing support and special friendship. Thanks as always, too, to Helen, Chris and Matthew Blackburn for their help and support.

Introduction

The adequacy of the cardiorespiratory system can generally be gauged from basic clinical signs such as heart rate, blood pressure, respiratory rate and depth, the skin's texture and colour, the use of accessory muscles of respiration and the patient's mental status. These basic signs should never be ignored but in critical illness, basic clinical assessment alone may be unreliable and misleading, therefore further monitoring techniques are usually required (Foxall, 2009).

Cardiac monitoring is essential when caring for the critically ill patient, as it provides highly valuable information. Abnormal cardiac rhythms can be recognised immediately, providing earlier diagnosis and therefore allowing quick and appropriate treatment (Jevon and Ewens, 2007). However, you should always remember that machines are fallible and only as safe as the person who is operating them! You must also remember that you should care for and treat the patient – not the machine!

There are hundreds of potential cardiac arrhythmias which is why this workbook considers the most common, important and potentially dangerous arrhythmias seen in the critically ill patient.

Many healthcare professionals find it difficult to get to grips with cardiac monitoring and arrhythmia recognition because it can be very complex and rather daunting. If you work your way through this book and carry out the exercises as you go, you will soon become more confident and competent at arrhythmia recognition and monitoring and will understand all the information on the subject that initially seems so complicated.

Here's to easy learning!

How to use this workbook

Accurate clinical assessment is particularly important in critically ill patients because haemodynamic status may change rapidly. Continuous cardiac monitoring will provide clear information that allows rapid adjustment of therapy (Jansen, 2002). This book is aimed at nurses working in critical care and high-dependency care areas, as well as other healthcare professionals who require an easy-to-understand introduction to cardiac arrhythmia recognition and management. It will provide a good foundation on which to build your knowledge.

If you are going to use a cardiac monitor, it is important to be able to interpret what you are seeing! So start at the beginning of the book, even if you feel quite happy about cardiac monitoring and arrhythmia recognition, because it will be good revision. Steadily work through the material, ensuring you understand all the information in each chapter before moving on to the next. Once you have read each chapter, complete the consolidation section to ensure you understand the information sufficiently. There is no specific consolidation section for Chapter 3; you will consolidate your learning from this chapter when you reach Chapter 5, where you can answer the questions and interpret the arrhythmias as you go. It will be good for you to find a mentor who will help you with any of the exercises you are unsure about.

If you don't know an answer or don't recognise an arrhythmia, try to work it out, based on the information you have already read. If you still can't, try discussing it with your chosen mentor. And if it is still not clear, then look up the answer in the answer section at the back of the book. Of course, if you do look up the answer, make sure you understand it – don't just accept it. If you have any problems, talk to your mentor. Use the answer section as a last resort and for checking purposes only! You'll learn far more by working things out for yourself. Those of you who already have a reasonable knowledge and understanding of cardiac monitoring and arrhythmia recognition, could attempt – if wished – the consolidation sections before reading the explanatory text. You will get a good idea of your current level of knowledge and be able to identify any gaps, which you can then concentrate on filling.

Aims of this workbook

The prime aim of this book is to extend your knowledge and clinical application of cardiac arrhythmia recognition.

After completing this workbook you will be able to:

- discuss the normal anatomy and physiology of the heart
- describe the principles of cardiac monitoring
- describe the normal ECG
- recognise common atrial, junctional and ventricular arrhythmias and atrioventricular blocks, state their effects on the body and what action should be taken – if any.

Management of the patient with life-threatening cardiac arrhythmias should always follow the Resuscitation Council (UK) guidelines and algorithms listed below.

- Adult Basic Life Support.
- AED Algorithm.
- In-Hospital Resuscitation.
- Adult Advanced Life Support.
- Adult Bradycardia Algorithm.
- Adult Tachycardia Algorithm.

These algorithms can be found at **http://www.resus.org.uk.**

Chapter 1

Anatomy and physiology of the heart

The cardiovascular system exists to provide tissue perfusion, to ensure the body's cells are provided with oxygen and nutrients at the same time as removing metabolic wastes (Gonce-Morton *et al.*, 2005).

Position of the heart

The heart can be described as a hollow organ located centrally in the chest directly behind the sternum, between the lungs, and it is a component of the mediastinum. It is supported at its base (which is at the *top*) by the great vessels and it rests on the diaphragm with its apex (which is at the *bottom*) directed anteriorly and to the left. Two-thirds of the mass of the heart lies to the left of the body's midline (Martini, 2006). See Fig. 1.1.

> **The heart provides the impetus to drive blood flow throughout the body.**

The function of the heart is to circulate blood and therefore oxygen and nutrients to the tissues; the blood then removes metabolic wastes from the tissues. It is a four-chambered double-pump. The **atria** receive returning blood and direct it to the ventricles. The **ventricles** provide the impetus to circulate the blood through the systemic and pulmonary circulations (Janson-Cohen, 2005).

The systemic and pulmonary circulation are illustrated in Fig. 1.2.

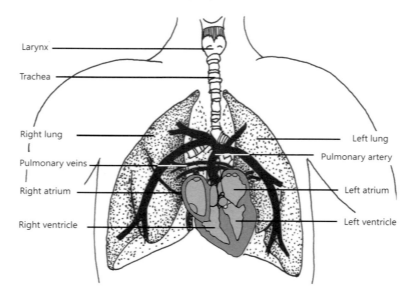

Fig. 1.1 *The heart in situ*

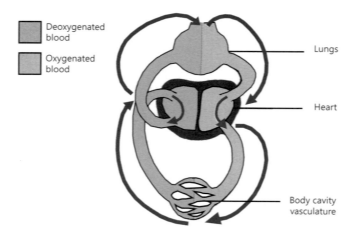

Fig. 1.2 *The systemic and pulmonary circulations*

The two sides of the heart are divided by the atrial and ventricular septa. The **atrial septum** is largely muscular tissue, and the **ventricular septum** is divided into two distinct parts – the membranous septum (the small, superior portion that borders the right atrium) and the larger muscular portion (which forms the true division between the left and right ventricles) as well as forming the wall of the left ventricle and functioning as part of the left ventricle (Marieb, 2006).

The heart wall

The heart consists of three distinct layers: the epicardium, the myocardium and the endocardium.

Epicardium

This is the thin, transparent layer of the heart wall. It also forms the visceral layer of the **pericardium,** which is made up of two sacs, an outer one consisting of fibrous tissue, and an inner one consisting of mucous membrane.

Myocardium

This is the middle layer and it is made of specialised cardiac muscle cells called **myocytes**. Cardiac muscle fibres (Fig. 1.3) are involuntary, striated and branched, arranged as interlacing bundles of fibres. They are responsible for cardiac contraction. Each cell has branches that lie in close relation to the next cell, forming junctions known as intercalated discs (Martini and Bartholomew, 2007). These fibres facilitate the passage of nervous impulses from one cell to the next, therefore each individual cell does not need its own nerve supply.

Endocardium

This is the inner layer. It is a membrane consisting of flattened squamous epithelial cells (Martini and Bartholomew, 2007) lining the inside of the myocardium and covering the heart valves and tendons.

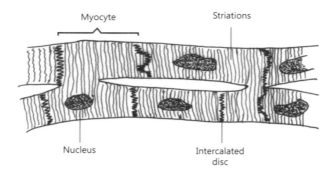

Fig. 1.3 *Cardiac muscle cell structure*

Heart valves

The heart valves comprise folds of fibrous tissue covered by endocardial tissue. They are anchored to the ventricular wall by the **chordae tendinae** at points where they meet the **papillary muscles**. Conmuscles opens the valve, and when they relax, the valve closes.

> **Heart valves allow one-way flow of blood from the atria into the ventricles and from the ventricles into the great vessels.**

There are four heart valves, namely the:

- **tricuspid valve** (the right atrioventricular valve)
- **pulmonary valve** (the outflow valve to the pulmonary artery)
- **mitral valve** (the left atrioventricular valve) and the
- **aortic valve** (the outflow valve to the aorta).

N.B. The pulmonary and aortic valves are also referred to as **semilunar** *valves.*

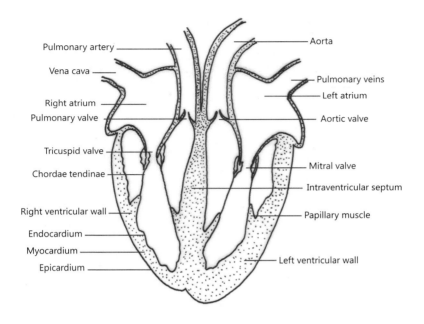

Fig. 1.4 *Sectional anatomy of the heart*

The blood flow through the heart is illustrated in Fig. 1.5 overpage and is described below.

(1) Superior and inferior **venae cavae** return deoxygenated blood from the systemic circulation to the **right atrium** from all areas of the body.

(2) Blood passes from the **right atrium** to the **right ventricle** via the tricuspid valve.

(3) Blood passes into the **pulmonary artery** via the pulmonary valve to the lungs where it picks up oxygen and releases carbon dioxide.

(4) Oxygenated blood returns to left side of the heart via the four **pulmonary veins**.

(5) Blood from the **left atrium** passes into the **left ventricle** via the mitral valve.

(6) Blood passes from the **left ventricle** into the **aorta** via the aortic valve to be distributed around the systemic circulation.

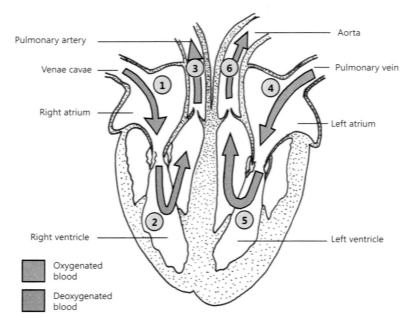

Fig. 1.5 *Blood flow through the heart (for more information see page 5)*

Blood supply to the heart

The heart requires a constant supply of oxygen and has its own circulation, which is known as the **coronary circulation**. The heart is supplied with arterial blood from the right and left coronary arteries. These are the first branches from the aorta immediately above the aortic valve (Janson-Cohen, 2005). The coronary arteries take 4% of the cardiac output from the left ventricle.

- **Right coronary artery:** this supplies the right atrium and ventricle.
- **Left coronary artery:** this subdivides into the circumflex artery, which supplies the left atrium and a portion of the left ventricle.
- **Anterior descending artery:** this is the other branch of the left coronary artery which supplies the remainder of the left ventricle and a small portion of the right ventricle (Mattson-Porth, 2005).

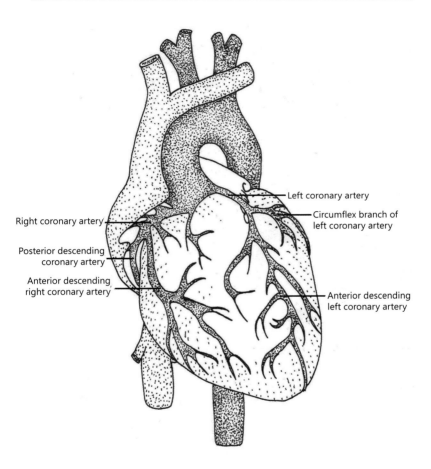

Fig. 1.6 *The coronary arteries*

As blood passes through the coronary circulation, it delivers oxygen and nutrients and collects carbon dioxide and other metabolic waste. The deoxygenated blood is drained back into the right atrium via the **coronary sinus**. The coronary sinus is a dilated vein that has no smooth muscle to alter its diameter (Janson-Cohen, 2005).

Conduction system of the heart

The heart's conduction system relies on the sinoatrial node (the pacemaker of the heart) and the atrioventricular node, which are small groups of specialised neuromuscular cells in the myocardium that *initiate* and then conduct electrical impulses over the heart muscle, causing it to contract.

These specialised cells have the ability to discharge electrical impulses automatically, that is without the influence of a nerve supply. This is known as **automaticity**. In other words, even if there is no stimulation from the central nervous system, the heart will continue to beat automatically (Mattson-Porth, 2005). However, the system can be stimulated or depressed by nerve impulses initiated from the brain (see page 13).

> **The lower down the conducting system the impulse is triggered, the slower the rate will be.**

There are two nodes that are central to the conduction process.:

First is the **sinoatrial (SA) node.** This small mass of specialised neuromuscular cells is located in the wall of the right atrium near the opening of the superior vena cava. The SA node is often described as the **pacemaker** of the heart because each heart beat is normally triggered by the impulses initiated by the SA node.

> **The sinoatrial node normally discharges at 60–100 beats per minute.**

The second is the **atrioventricular (AV) node.** This mass of specialised neuromuscular cells is situated in the wall of the atrial septum near the atrioventricular valves. Normally the AV node is stimulated by the wave of electrical impulses initiated by the SA node, sweeping over the atrial myocardium via **internodal** tracts or pathways.

However, it is also capable of initiating electrical impulses if there is no stimulation from the SA node or the central nervous system.

> **The atrioventricular node normally discharges at 40–60 beats per minute.**

The **bundle of His** (also called the atrioventricular or AV bundle) consists of a mass of specialised neuromuscular fibres originating from the AV node and passing downwards in the septum that separates the left and right ventricles. This bundle of fibres then divides into two branches, one feeding each ventricle – these are the **left and right bundle branches**. Within the myocardium of the ventricles, the branches further divide into a network of fine filaments called the **Purkinje fibres** (or fibres of Purkinje). The bundle of His and the Purkinje fibres (together referred to as the **His–Purkinje** fibres) convey electrical impulses from the AV node to the myocardium of the ventricles.

> **The His–Purkinje fibres normally discharge at 20–40 beats per minute.**

The electrical impulses initiated by the SA node stimulate the atrial myocardium to contract. This first wave of impulses and contraction stimulate the AV node to continue the wave of contraction to the apex of the heart via the His–Purkinje fibres and then upward over the myocardium. In this way, the ventricular wave of contraction begins at the apex of the heart (at the bottom) and blood is forced upward into the pulmonary artery and aorta to leave the heart at its base (at the top) (Martini, 2006).

The function of the **bundle branches** is to conduct unified electrical impulses throughout the ventricles, thus causing brief, powerful and unified contraction of the ventricles.

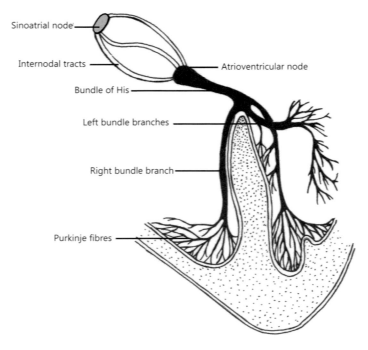

Fig. 1.7 *The conduction system of the heart*

The cardiac cycle

The cardiac cycle is a series of pressure changes, valve actions and electrical potentials (see Chapter 2) that bring about movement of blood through the heart during one complete heart beat (Bruck *et al.*, 2005).

Think of it in three distinct phases:

- Atrial systole.
- Ventricular systole.
- Ventricular diastole.

Phase 1: Atrial systole

As blood is drained from the superior and inferior venae cavae into the right atrium, and from the pulmonary veins into the left atrium, **atrial pressure** rises. During this period the atrioventricular valves are closed. Towards the end of atrial filling the ventricles start to relax so that **ventricular pressure** falls.

When atrial pressure *exceeds* ventricular pressure, the atrioventricular valves are pushed open. Around 70–80% of the blood then flows *passively* from the atria into the ventricles. As blood leaves the atria, the pressure falls and when the atria contract, the remaining blood is forced into the ventricles. This is known as **atrial kick**.

Phase 2: Ventricular systole

Ventricular systole (contraction) follows atrial systole. **Ventricular pressure** exceeds **atrial pressure** and causes the AV valves to close. The ventricle is now full of blood and both the AV valves and semilunar valves are closed.

The ventricles contract and ventricular pressure rises until it exceeds that in the aorta and pulmonary artery. This forces open the pulmonary and aortic valves and blood flows into the pulmonary artery and aorta. The time taken from myocardial contraction to the ejection of blood into the circulation is known as the **ejection period**.

Phase 3: Ventricular diastole

At the end of ventricular systole, the ventricles begin to relax. Ventricular pressure then *decreases* and arterial pressure *increases*, causing a backflow of blood towards the ventricles and forcing the aortic and pulmonary valves to close.

Ventricular diastole occurs, during which time the SA node initiates the next impulse and the beginning of another cardiac cycle.

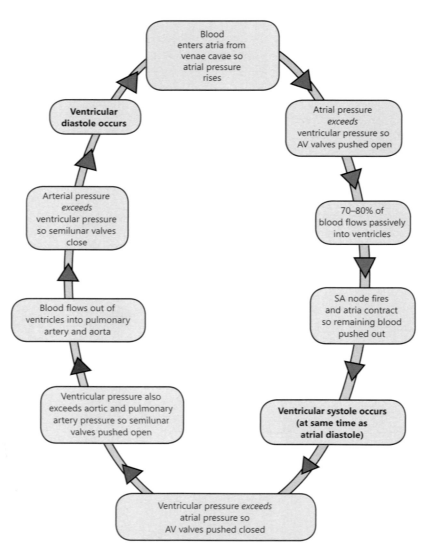

Fig. 1.8 *The cardiac cycle*

Nerve supply to the heart

In addition to the intrinsic stimulation of the myocardium (automaticity) as described above, the heart is influenced by nerves that originate in the **cardiac centre** within the **medulla oblongata** of the brain.

The cardiac centre has two distinct parts – inhibitory and excitatory. The nerves originating from the cardiac centre are part of the **parasympathetic** (inhibitory) and **sympathetic** (excitatory) nervous systems and work antagonistically (that is, against each other) (Martini, 2006).

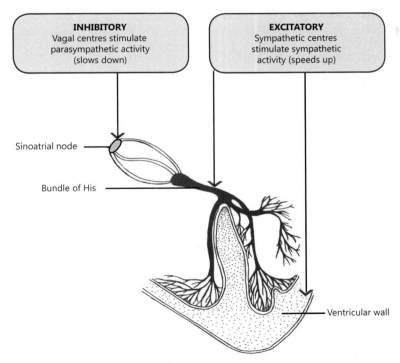

Fig. 1.9 *Nerve supply to the heart*

> **Sympathetic system**
>
> **This acts most strongly when you are in danger.
> It comes out in** *sympathy* **with you and increases the body's
> effectiveness so that you can escape danger
> (the 'fight or flight' response).**
>
> **Parasympathetic system**
> **This does the opposite: it calms and relaxes.**

The **vagus nerve** supplies the heart and is part of the parasympathetic nervous system.

• The **parasympathetic** system tends to *slow* the rate at which the SA node fires impulses, therefore *decreasing* the rate and force of contraction.

• The **sympathetic** system tends to *speed up* the rate of impulse production from the SA node, thus *increasing* the rate and force of contraction.

The rate at which the heart beats and the force of its contraction are a fine balance of the effects of the parasympathetic and sympathetic systems. Heart rate is usually decreased during rest and increased during excitement and exercise and when the blood volume is decreased.

Other factors influencing heart rate

Baroreceptors

These also connect with the cardiac centre and are sensitive to pressure within the blood vessels. Any increase in blood pressure will stimulate the baroreceptors, which in turn stimulate the cardiac inhibitory centre. This stimulation increases vagal tone and brings about a reduction in heart rate, therefore reducing cardiac output and thus blood pressure (Foxall, 2009).

Adrenaline (epinephrine) and noradrenaline (norepinephrine)

Heart rate is increased by the release of these hormones from the adrenal glands.

Breathing

Deep breathing increases vagal tone, that is it stimulates the vagus nerve (parasympathetic) and therefore reduces heart rate.

Oxygen

Hypoxia and hypercarbia decrease vagal tone, allowing sympathetic impulses to become dominant, so increasing the heart rate.

Body temperature

This affects the cardiac centre and a rise in temperature increases the heart rate.

Thyroxine

This thyroid hormone directly affects the SA node and heart rate increases.

Consolidation

See pages 137–138 for answers

1.1 What is the function of the heart?

_____

1.2 Describe the position of the heart and its gross anatomy.

_____

_____

_____

1.3 Label this diagram of the heart.

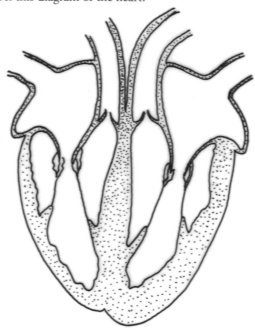

1.4   What are the three layers of the heart called?

_____

_____

1.5   Outline the main features of a cardiac muscle cell.

_____

_____

_____

1.6   Name the heart valves and their positions within the heart.

_____

_____

_____

_____

1.7   Describe how blood flows through the heart.

_____

_____

_____

_____

1.8   Describe the coronary circulation.

_____

_____

_____

1.9   Label this diagram of the conducting system of the heart.

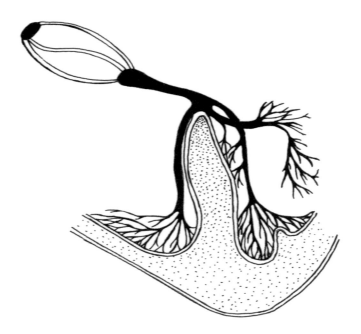

1.10   At what rate does the SA node normally discharge?

1.11   At what rate does the AV node normally discharge?

_____

1.12   At what rate do the His–Purkinje fibres normally discharge?

_____

1.13   Briefly describe the cardiac cycle.

_____

_____

_____

_____

_____

1.14   Briefly describe the nerve supply to the heart.

_____

_____

1.15   Other than the nerve supply, what other factors influence heart rate?

_____

_____

_____

_____

Notes

Chapter 2

Principles of cardiac monitoring and the normal ECG

Cardiac monitoring is used to pick up the electrical signals generated by the heart and to display them as a continuous trace – the electrocardiogram (ECG). The ECG does not pick up mechanical activity (i.e. the extent of contraction) and of course there can be electrical activity with no mechanical activity (Levine *et al.*, 2008).

> **Cardiac monitoring should be used in any situation in which the patient is at risk of developing cardiac arrhythmias.**

Methods of monitoring

There are three methods of cardiac monitoring:

• **Continuous monitoring:** essential for all critically ill patients but should only be used to gain information about the patient's heart rate and rhythm.
• **12-lead ECG:** used for precise diagnosis of cardiac problems.
• **Defibrillator paddles:** used in emergency situations only.

One of the most important things to remember is that if you monitor 10 people who are all in sinus rhythm (the normal rhythm of the heart) the resulting traces will all look a bit different! Therefore:

> **You need to observe for the *characteristics* of the waveform.**

Electrode positioning and lead selection

There is much debate about the importance of precisely how electrodes are placed and the selection of leads. What everyone agrees is important is that the electrode gel does not *dry out!* As a general rule place the electrodes thus (Fig. 2.1) (Cowley, 2006):

- **red** wire (positive lead) on the right shoulder
- **yellow** wire (negative lead) on the left shoulder
- **green** or **black** wire (ground lead) at the apex of the heart.

This placement (Fig. 2.1) gives a general triangular shape with the electrodes close enough to the heart to pick up a good signal but far enough away should chest compression or defibrillation be required. The number of leads varies for differing monitoring systems inasmuch as there can be three, four or five leads. Follow your local policy for lead placement.

When monitoring heart rhythm, getting a good signal is more important than the precise placement of the electrodes. Generally for monitoring rhythm, lead II is used but – in practice – you need to monitor with the lead that gives the clearest display (Cowley, 2006). The lead used to monitor heart rhythm is selected on the cardiac monitor.

There is also some controversy about whether to place the electrodes over bone or muscle. Bone is not as good a conductor as muscle is, which therefore favours muscle, however muscle tends to produce more interference (Cowley, 2006) so generally, therefore, electrodes are placed over *bone* (Jevon and Ewens, 2007).

> **When you change the electrodes make sure you are consistent in their positioning.**
>
> **(Remember, they should be changed every 24 hours.)**

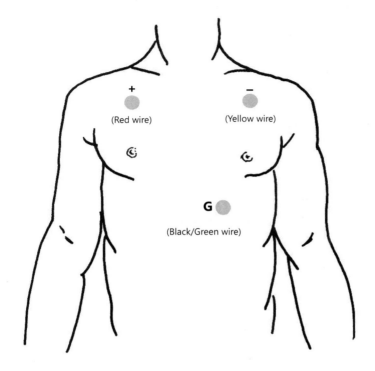

Fig. 2.1 *Electrode placement*

ECG paper

ECG paper allows the waveforms produced by the heart's electrical activity to be recorded using a stylus (or pen).

The squares on the paper allow you to determine both the time and the amplitude of the heart's electrical activity, as set out in Fig. 2.2 overpage.

On ECG paper:

- The *horizontal* axis represents time in seconds.
- The *vertical* axis represents amplitude in millivolts (mV).

The ECG machine is usually run at a speed of 25 mm per second (Davis, 2005).

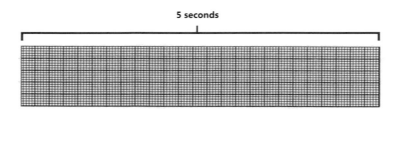

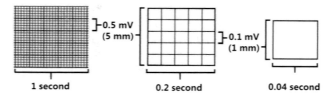

Fig. 2.2 *ECG paper and associated timings*

The set-up of cardiac monitoring equipment and managing the patient is summarised in Table 2.1. Table 2.2 lists typical problems encountered during cardiac monitoring, some of which are illustrated in Figs 2.3–2.7.

Table 2.1 Setting up cardiac monitoring equipment and managing the patient

Action	Rationale
Clearly explain to the patient what you are going to do and why (and explain that he or she may hear alarms – but should not be alarmed!)	To gain consent and cooperation and to reduce anxiety
Ensure the patient's skin is clean and dry, using an alcohol swab on oily skin if necessary (clip or shave any excess hair if necessary)	To ensure electrodes stay in place and good electrical contact is made to get an accurate trace
Switch on the monitor and select monitoring lead II unless advised otherwise	Lead II is the most commonly used for monitoring (Jevon and Ewens, 2007)
If the electrodes are the press-stud type, attach the leads to the electrodes before applying them to the patient's skin	To avoid pressing hard on the patient's chest (it is uncomfortable for the patient and you will lose electrode contact)
Ensure the monitor can be clearly seen and that the ECG trace is clear	To maintain patient safety
Frequently observe the monitor for changes in rate and rhythm	To maintain patient safety
Alter the gain (which increases or decreases the size of the trace) if necessary	To ensure an accurate trace (it can be misinterpreted if the size is inappropriate)
Verify that you have an appropriate ECG trace by ensuring it corresponds with the patient's apical rate (Levine et al., 2008)	To ensure accurate readings
Set the monitor alarms to appropriate levels according to the patient's clinical condition (usually 10–20 bpm above and below the patient's heart rate)	To maintain patient safety
If possible, print a rhythm strip and document this in the patient's notes	To provide a baseline rhythm for future comparison
Document any changes and inform senior or medical staff of any concerns	To maintain patient safety
Ensure the gel on all electrodes remains moist and change electrodes every 24 hours	To ensure the electrode gel does not dry out and ensure accurate readings

Table 2.2 Problems encountered during cardiac monitoring

Problem	Likely causes	What do to about it
Wandering baseline (Fig. 2.3)	• Patient's breathing movements • Patient moving excessively • Electrodes not applied correctly	• Make sure electrodes are not on lower ribs • Encourage patient to remain calm and still • Replace electrodes
Artefact/ interference (Fig. 2.4)	• Patient shivering • Interference from other electrical equipment • Electrodes not applied correctly • Worn wires or cables	• Keep patient warm • Move other equipment as far away from patient as possible • Replace electrodes • Replace appropriate wires, cables or monitor
No waveform (flat trace) (Fig. 2.5)	• Asystole (eliminate this possibility) • Electrodes have become disconnected • ECG gain set too low • Monitor leads are disconnected • Electrode gel dried out • Worn wires or cables	• Check the patient immediately, summon help and commence cardiopulmonary resuscitation if asystole present • Replace electrodes • Increase gain • Reconnect leads • Replace electrodes • Replace appropriate wires, cables or monitor
False low reading (Fig. 2.6)	• ECG complexes too small due to weak signal • Electrodes not applied correctly • Worn wires or cables	• Increase gain • Replace electrodes • Replace appropriate wires, cables or monitor
False high reading (Fig. 2.7)	• Gain set too high • Electrodes not applied correctly	• Reduce gain • Replace electrodes
Frequent alarming but patient is OK	• Alarm levels set too high or too low	• Alter the alarm parameters to an appropriate level. However, never turn off an alarm until you know the reason • If in doubt – SHOUT!
Faulty equipment	• Worn wires or cables • Poor grounding	• Do not use faulty components as they could give an electric shock to the patient • Get a new monitor!

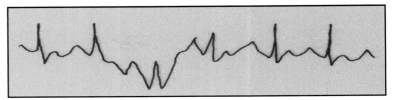

Fig. 2.3 *Wandering baseline*

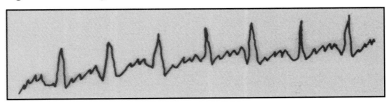

Fig. 2.4 *Artefact/interference*

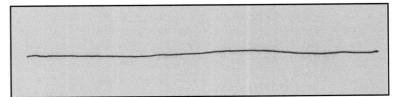

Fig. 2.5 *Flat trace*

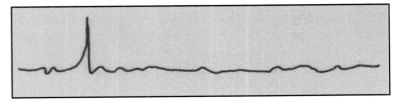

Fig. 2.6 *False low reading*

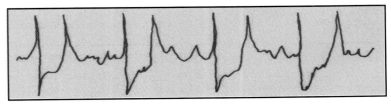

Fig. 2.7 *False high reading*

Electrophysiology of depolarisation and repolarisation

Without an electrical stimulus, the heart would not beat. The heart has specialised cells with four characteristics that ensure the heart continues to pump with or without stimulation from the central nervous system (Levine *et al.*, 2008). These are:

1. **Automaticity** (spontaneous initiation of an electrical impulse).

2. **Excitability** (the cells respond to an electrical stimulus as a result of electrolyte shifts).

3. **Conductivity** (the electrical impulse is transmitted from one cell to the next).

4. **Contractility** (the cell contracts as a result of an electrical stimulus).

There are two types of cardiac muscle cells, namely **contractile** and **non-contractile** cells. The *contractile* cells make up 99% of all cardiac muscle cells and provide the powerful contraction that propels blood around the body (Martini and Bartholemew, 2007). The conducting system, which initiates and controls those contractions, is made up of *non-contractile* cells.

The human body contains various electrolytes in solution through which electrical currents will flow. In the heart, each cardiac cell contains such electrolyte fluids and is also surrounded by them. The main electrolytes responsible for electrical activity within the heart are sodium (Na^+), potassium (K^+) and calcium (Ca^{++}) (Davis, 2005). In resting (or polarised) cardiac cells, the inside of the cell is relatively negatively charged in comparison to the outside of the cell, which is positively charged; this creates what is known as the **resting potential**.

When myocardial cells are stimulated by an electrical impulse, a change takes place in the cell membrane's permeability and various electrolytes move across the cell membrane by diffusion or active transport so that the inside of the cell becomes positively charged.

The process by which the inside of a cell becomes more positive in relation to the outside is called **depolarisation** and it is this movement of electrolytes that generates the electrical flow, which is picked up by the ECG. This is known as the **action potential** (Fig. 2.8).

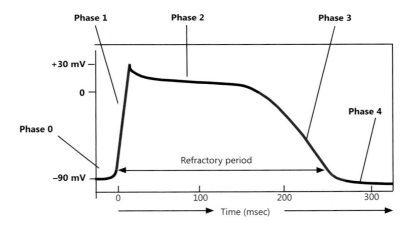

Fig. 2.8 *The action potential*

There are five phases of the action potential.

Phase 0—Rapid depolarisation

This happens because positively charged sodium and calcium move into the cell. Sodium moves in rapidly and calcium more slowly, through slow calcium channels. The inside of the cell therefore becomes more positively charged.

Phase 1—Early repolarisation

The sodium channels close so no more sodium can enter the cell. Therefore the inside of the cell cannot become any more positively charged.

Phase 2—Plateau phase

Calcium continues to flow in slowly, whilst positively charged potassium starts to flow out of the cell, so the overall charge starts to become more negative.

Phase 3—Rapid repolarisation

The calcium channels close, so no more calcium enters the cell and potassium flows out rapidly, so the inside of the cell becomes more negative more quickly.

Phase 4—Resting phase

The sodium, potassium and calcium return to their original state.

A **depolarised** cell (as shown in Fig. 2.9) is electrically negative on the outside compared with any of its neighbouring non-stimulated cells. A potential difference therefore exists *between* the cells and a current flows between them until they have all been depolarised.

When the cell is depolarised it becomes *excited* and ready for *action*. It also stimulates the cell or cells next to it so there is a smooth wave of depolarisation all the way down the conducting tissue of the heart.

The refractory period

The refractory period is how long it takes for an excitable membrane that has returned to its resting state following excitation to be ready for a second stimulus. See also Fig. 2.8 on the previous page.

During the so-called *relative* **refractory period**, it is possible for a very strong electrical impulse to depolarise the cell early.

During the *absolute* **refractory period**, the cells cannot be stimulated at all.

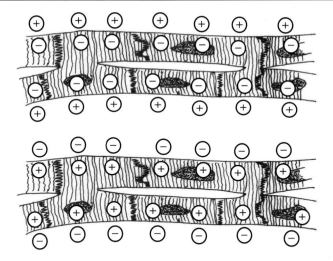

Fig. 2.9 *Polarised (resting) cardiac muscle cells* (upper panel) *and depolarised cardiac cells* (lower panel)

A single heart beat

Each beat of the heart is initiated by the SA node. On the ECG trace it is made up of a normal P wave, a QRS complex and a T wave (Fig. 2.10).

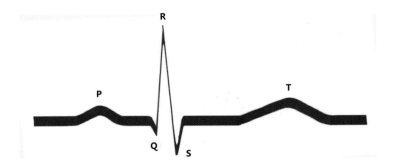

Fig. 2.10 *One heart beat*

The rhythm should be regular with a rate of approximately 72 beats per minute (b.p.m.). When this is the case, the heart is said to be in **sinus rhythm** (Fig. 2.11), which is the normal rhythm of the heart.

If there is *any* deviation from this sinus rhythm, an arrhythmia is present.

You will not be able to recognise an arrhythmia if you cannot first recognise normal sinus rhythm, as this is the rhythm against which all other rhythms are compared (Levine *et al.*, 2008).

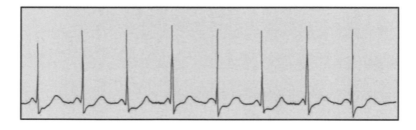

Fig. 2.11 *Sinus rhythm*

Note that the heart can be regular in rhythm with a rate of 72 b.p.m. and *not be* sinus in nature.

You must therefore be able to recognise the normal characteristics of the P wave, the QRS complex, the T wave and intervals and segments.

Now read on ...

Waveforms

There are four stages within each heart beat and each is represented in terms of waves, namely the P, Q, R, S and T waves.

Stage 1 – Sinoatrial node impulse

The SA node fires an electrical impulse, which spreads over the atria via the internodal tracts, resulting in atrial depolarisation. This is denoted by the *P wave*. Depolarisation causes the atria to contract.

The P wave is 0.06–0.12 seconds in duration.

Stage 2 – Atrial repolarisation

There is atrial repolarisation (i.e. the atria relax). However, the wave of repolarisation is usually not seen as it is hidden by the more powerful QRS complex.

Stage 3 – Ventricular depolarisation

Ventricular depolarisation occurs next as the wave of depolarisation passes down the bundle of His, the right and left bundle branches and the Purkinje fibres. It is represented by the QRS complex. Ventricular depolarisation causes the ventricles to contract.

The QRS complex should last for less than 0.12 seconds and is measured from the beginning of the *Q wave* to the end of the *S wave*.

Remember, all three waves (Q, R and S) may not be present because of the speed of contraction, but the heart's activity can still be normal.

Stage 4 – Ventricular repolarisation

Ventricular repolarisation is represented by the *T wave* as the myocardial cells return to their resting charge.

Intervals and segments

Intervals *contain* waves. **Segments** are the lines *between* the waves where there is no electrical activity and the trace does not deflect either above or below the baseline (i.e. they are **isoelectric**) (Viney, 1999).

The intervals and segments in one heart beat are shown in Fig. 2.12.

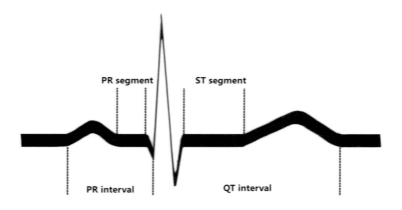

Fig. 2.12 *Intervals and segments in one heart beat*

PR interval

The PR interval is the time from the beginning of the P wave to the beginning of the QRS complex. It indicates the time taken for the impulse to pass from the SA node to the ventricles (Levine *et al.*, 2008). It therefore reflects atrial *depolarisation* and is between 0.12 and 0.2 seconds in duration.

• A *long* PR interval may indicate that there is a conduction delay through the atria or AV node.

• A *short* PR interval suggests the impulse originated away from the SA node (Viney, 1999).

PR segment

The PR segment indicates the time between the end of the P wave and the beginning of the QRS complex (Davis, 2005).

ST segment

The ST segment indicates the time between the end of the S wave and the beginning of the T wave and represents the beginning of ventricular repolarisation. The beginning of the ST segment is known as the J point (Levine *et al.*, 2008). The ST segment should be isoelectric and if it is raised or depressed it may indicate the presence of myocardial ischaemia.

QT interval

The QT interval represents the time from the beginning of the Q wave to the end of the T wave and therefore reflects the time taken for the ventricles to depolarise and repolarise. It usually lasts for 0.36–0.44 seconds.

Deflections

The choice of electrode position will dictate the **morphology** of the ECG complex that appears on the monitor.

Remember that depolarisation is a wave of *positive* charges flowing through the heart muscle. If the wave of depolarisation is flowing towards a *positive* electrode, then the result will be a *positive* morphology (an upstroke) of the ECG.

When monitoring using lead II (see page 22) with the electrodes placed in the position shown in Fig. 2.1, the deflection of the waveforms goes in the *opposite* direction to the wave of depolarisation.

As the impulse is travelling from negative to positive poles and the wave of depolarisation passes downwards over the atria, there is a positive (*upward*) deflection on the ECG – this is the *P wave*.

Then there is an isoelectric (flat) portion where there is no electrical activity. This is the *PR segment*, just before the *QRS complex*.

The *Q wave* is slightly negative (downward) and, as the impulse spreads over the bundle of His and passes down the bundle branches, there is a downward wave of depolarisation, so the *R wave* is positive.

The impulse then passes along the fibres of Purkinje and upwards over the ventricles, so the *S wave* is negative. This is followed by repolarisation reflected by the isoelectric *ST segment* and the *T wave*.

> **A deeply negative Q wave is indicative of previous myocardial ischaemia.**

The deflections in one heart beat are shown in Fig. 2.13.

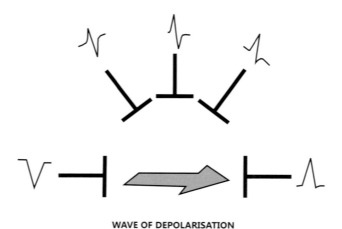

WAVE OF DEPOLARISATION

Fig. 2.13 *The deflections in one heart beat*

Consolidation

See pages 139–142 for answers

2.1   What is the purpose of cardiac monitoring?

_____

_____

2.2   Does the ECG pick up the mechanical activity of the heart?

_____

2.3   Name three methods of cardiac monitoring.

_____

_____

2.4   Generally, where should the electrodes be placed?

_____

_____

2.5   Which lead is generally used for monitoring?

_____

2.6   Why are the electrodes usually placed over bone?

_____

_____

2.7   What amount of time is represented by one of the very small squares on the ECG paper?

_____

2.8   What amount of time is represented by one small square on the ECG paper?

_____

2.9   What amount of time is represented by one large square on the ECG paper?

_____

2.10   What are the main considerations when caring for a patient who is undergoing cardiac monitoring?

_____

_____

_____

_____

_____

_____

_____

_____

_____

2.11   What are the causes and what would be your action if there is a wandering baseline?

_____

_____

2.12   What are the causes and what would be your action if there is artefact/interference on the monitor?

_____

_____

2.13   What are the causes and what would be your action if there is no waveform, only a flat trace?

_____

_____

_____

2.14   What are the causes and what would be your action if there is a false low reading?

_____

_____

2.15   What are the causes and what would be your action if there is a false high reading?

_____

_____

2.16   What are the causes and what would be your action if the monitor is frequently alarming?

_____

_____

2.17   What would be your action if the monitor is faulty?

_____

2.18   What are the four characteristics of cardiac cells that ensure the heart continues to pump with or without central nervous stimulation?

_____

2.19   What are the two types of cardiac muscle cells?

_____

2.20   What type of cardiac muscle cells make up the conducting system of the heart?

_____

2.21   What three main electrolytes are responsible for electrical activity in the heart?

_____

2.22   Within a polarised cardiac muscle cell, is the charge negative or positive?

_____

_____

2.23   What happens when an electrical impulse stimulates a polarised myocardial cell?

_____

_____

_____

2.24   How many phases are there in an action potential?

_____

_____

2.25   Name the phases of the action potential.

_____

_____

2.26   What is the difference between the _relative_ refractory period and the _absolute_ refractory period?

_____

_____

2.27   What name is given to the change by which the inside of a cell becomes more positive in relation to the outside?

_____

2.28   Is a depolarised cell electrically negative or positive on the outside?

_____

2.29   What characteristics define sinus rhythm?

_____

_____

_____

2.30   What are the four main stages of one heart beat?

_____

_____

_____

2.31   What does the P wave represent?

_____

2.32   What does the QRS complex represent?

_____

2.33   What does the T wave represent?

_____

|_____

2.34   What is the difference between intervals and segments on the ECG?

_____

_____

2.35   Label the waves on the following diagram.

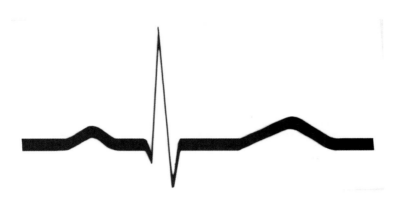

2.36   What does the PR interval denote?

_____

2.37   What does the PR segment denote?

_____

2.38   What does the ST segment denote?

_____

2.39   What does the QT interval denote?

_____

2.40   Label the intervals and segments on the following diagram.

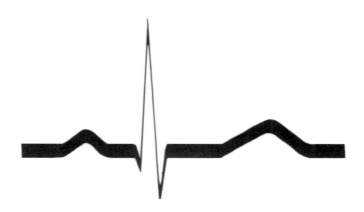

2.41   If lead II is being used, would the ECG deflection travel in the *same* direction or the *opposite* direction to that of the wave of depolarisation?

_____

2.42   Under the supervision of your mentor, set up and attach a cardiac monitor to a patient, following local procedure. Discuss your findings with your mentor and record them in the table below.

	Date	Comments and observations	Signature of mentor
1			
2			

	Date	Comments and observations	Signature of mentor
3			
4			

Notes

Chapter 3

Recognising common arrhythmias

There are literally hundreds of different types of cardiac arrhythmias (Jaeger, 2008). Therefore, in this chapter we will consider the most common arrhythmias you are likely to encounter in a critical care or high-dependency environment.

Cardiac arrhythmias are very common and produce symptoms such as dizziness, palpitations and syncope. They are generally benign (Jaeger, 2008) although, in a critically ill patient they can create further complications for the patient with an already compromised cardiovascular system.

In addition to these relatively benign arrhythmias, there are arrhythmias that are dangerous for the patient if they are left untreated and there are arrhythmias that bring about sudden death! The cardiac monitor can give you prior warning of problems that may lie ahead, many of which can be resolved or abated to some degree.

Classification of arrhythmias

Cardiac arrhythmias are generally classified by their site of origin (Haworth *et al.*, 2004), for example SA node (sinus rhythms), atrial (supraventricular), junctional or ventricular arrhythmias.

These arrhythmias result from a disturbance in **impulse formation** (Jevon and Ewens, 2007). However, **heart blocks** result from a disturbance in **impulse conduction** (Jevon and Ewens, 2007).

Cardiac arrhythmias may arise for several reasons:

1. From **abnormal electrical conduction** within the heart.

2. Through **re-entry circuits** whereby an impulse travels where it has already been.

3. From **enhanced automaticity** (an irritable focus within the conducting system firing an impulse when it shouldn't).

(Haworth *et al.*, 2004)

The general management of arrhythmias will be covered within this chapter, but for a more comprehensive description see Chapter 4.

SINUS NODE ARRHYTHMIAS

Sinus arrhythmia

In sinus arrhythmia (Fig. 3.1) the heart rate stays within *normal* limits but it is irregular. The rhythm generally corresponds to the respiratory cycle, increasing during inspiration and decreasing during expiration, because of the effect breathing has on the vagus nerve (see Fig. 3.2).

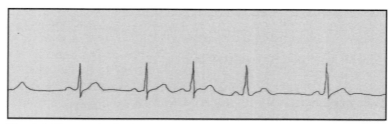

Fig. 3.1 *Sinus arrhythmia*

The P wave, QRS complex and T wave are normal but the RR intervals are irregular. It is usually insignificant and requires no treatment but it may be indicative of a more serious problem.

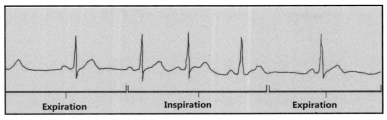

Fig. 3.2 *Sinus arrhythmia relating to respiratory cycle*

CAUSES OF SINUS ARRHYTHMIA

Sick sinus syndrome

Digoxin toxicity

Myocardial infarction

Raised intracranial pressure

Management

Sinus arrhythmia often occurs naturally in children and athletes. Unless the patient is symptomatic, it is no cause for concern and requires no treatment. If sinus arrhythmia has an underlying cause (such as those listed above) it should be closely monitored and the cause dealt with swiftly.

Sinus bradycardia

Sinus bradycardia (Fig. 3.3) has a regular rhythm and a rate of less than 60 beats per minute. The P wave, QRS complex and T wave are normal.

It often occurs in athletes and during relaxation and sleep when the body's metabolic demands are reduced. There is no cause for concern. However, if the patient has an underlying condition, a decrease in cardiac output may occur – resulting in hypotension – and the patient may be predisposed to further serious arrhythmias.

A bradycardia of less than 45 b.p.m. is not well tolerated and will produce symptoms of reduced cardiac output.

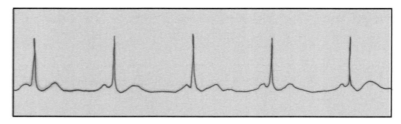

Fig. 3.3 *Sinus bradycardia*

CAUSES OF SINUS BRADYCARDIA

Increased vagal stimulation caused e.g. by sleep, vomiting, carotid sinus massage, inferior myocardial infarction, pneumothorax

Raised intracranial pressure

Hypothermia

Late hypovolaemia

Hypoxia

Acidosis

Electrolyte disturbances

Some drugs
(e.g. digoxin, calcium-channel blockers, beta-blockers)

Management

For as long as the patient is asymptomatic, no treatment is necessary. However, if the patient is compromised by the bradycardia, swift treatment is necessary. A heart rate of less than 60 b.p.m. may cause the patient to collapse or suffer symptoms of inadequate perfusion, particularly if there is a sudden bradycardia – in which case the adult bradycardia algorithm should be used (Resuscitation Council UK, 2009). Assess airway, breathing and circulation (ABC), ensure the patient's airway is clear, and give them oxygen and respiratory assistance if required.

Transcutaneous or transvenous pacing may be required with drug intervention to support the patient's circulation prior to pacing (e.g. using atropine and/or inotropic agents).

Sinus tachycardia

Sinus tachycardia has a regular rhythm. The P waves, QRS complexes and T waves are normal and regular with a rate of 100–160 b.p.m.

In sustained sinus tachycardia, the P waves may increase in amplitude or be superimposed on the preceding T wave, sometimes making identification difficult.

CAUSES OF SINUS TACHYCARDIA

Strenuous exercise

Anxiety

Haemorrhage

Hypovolaemia

Pain

Acute myocardial infarction

Initial stage of cardiogenic shock

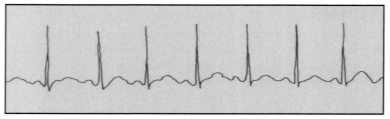

Fig. 3.4 *Sinus tachycardia*

Sinus tachycardia is of little or no significance when there is no underlying cause or it occurs as a response to strenuous exercise or a high-anxiety state. In the critically ill patient, it may be caused by pain and/or hypovolaemia for which treatment should be given swiftly. Sinus tachycardia can have serious consequences as it increases cardiac work and therefore oxygen consumption and can therefore lead to heart failure. In patients with underlying heart disease, it can be an ominous prognostic sign.

Management

If there is no underlying cause, the tachycardia is transient, and the patient is asymptomatic, no treatment is necessary – but the patient should be observed. With a sustained sinus tachycardia, however, even if the patient is asymptomatic, the cause should be determined and treated. Sinus tachycardia can severely reduce cardiac output because of the reduction in ventricular filling time, so there is less blood in the ventricles to pump into the circulation. In addition to this, the heart has to work harder as it tries to maintain the circulation and therefore it needs more oxygen (which it cannot get because of the reduction in cardiac output) which is why this chain of events can lead to heart failure. Symptoms of reduced cardiac output are produced and treatment should be instigated to slow the heart rate and increase the power of ventricular contraction.

Here are the most common treatments:

• For tachycardia caused by *haemorrhage* or *hypovolaemia* – stop the bleeding and replace fluid.

• For tachycardia with another cause, give beta-adrenergic blockers and/or calcium-channel blockers.

In the critically ill patient it may also be necessary to support the circulation with **inotropic** agents to increase cardiac contractility, which will increase blood pressure and improve oxygen delivery to the tissues.

ATRIAL (SUPRAVENTRICULAR) ARRHYTHMIAS

Premature atrial contractions (PACs)

Premature atrial contractions are also known as atrial premature beats (APBs) or atrial ectopic beats. They are simply beats that occur sooner than the expected beat. They occur because an irritable focus outside of the SA node fires, causing the heart to contract. It takes a little time for the SA node to reset itself so there is a slight pause before the next beat, although this is not long enough to be a full compensatory pause. PACs occur in patients with underlying heart disease but they also occur quite normally and cause no problems in people who are disease free.

CAUSES OF PREMATURE ATRIAL CONTRACTIONS

Smoking

Alcohol consumption

Exhaustion

Caffeine consumption

Pyrexia

Infection

Coronary heart disease

Valvular disease

Lung disease

Hypoxia

Respiratory failure

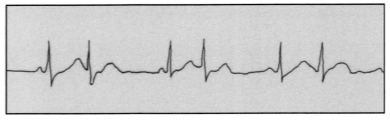

Fig. 3.5 *Premature atrial contractions*

In patients with an underlying cardiac problem they can lead to further arrhythmias or heart failure or to symptoms of a reduced cardiac output (if the PACs are frequent). They therefore need to be closely monitored and treatment should be instigated where necessary.

Management

If the patient has no cardiac disease and is asymptomatic, treatment is rarely necessary. If the PACs are caused by a removable cause such as caffeine, alcohol or other such irritants, then the patient should be advised to reduce intake of such substances. In patients who have an underlying disease with symptoms resuling from the PACs, drug treatment may be commenced to increase the atrial refractory period (e.g. digoxin).

Atrial flutter

Atrial flutter is a form of supraventricular tachycardia. It is present when there is an irritable focus within the atria firing at a rate of approximately 300 b.p.m. Not all of these impulses pass through the AV node but when one does, the ventricles contract. So the atrial rate is much higher than the ventricular rate. P waves are not distinguishable and it is recognised by a typical so-called saw-toothed appearance, caused by the flutter waves. The flutter originates from a single focus within the atria. If it takes two impulses (flutter waves) to stimulate ventricular contraction; the conduction ratio is 2:1 three flutter waves; 3:1 four flutter waves; 4:1 ... and so on. A 2:1 block is most common and you will see an atrial rate of approximately 300 b.p.m. with a ventricular rate of approximately 150 b.p.m.

CAUSES OF ATRIAL FLUTTER

Hypoxia

Acute myocardial infarction

Cardiac surgery

Valvular disease

Chronic obstructive pulmonary disease

Infection

Hypovolaemia

It is referred to as a 'block' because the AV node 'blocks' half of the impulses and they do not pass through the node. The QRS complex is generally normal and the T wave is not identifiable.

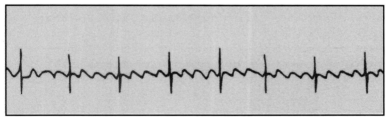

Fig. 3.6 *Atrial flutter*

Management

If the ventricular rate is normal, the patient may be asymptomatic, but if the ventricular rate is badly affected and is too slow or too high, symptoms of reduced cardiac output and perfusion disturbances will be seen. The goals of treatment are:

- To control the ventricular rate.
- To restore sinus rhythm.
- To prevent recurrences of atrial flutter.

If the patient is unstable, synchronous direct-current (DC) cardioversion is commonly the initial treatment of choice (see Chapter 5). An antiarrhythmic agent, beta-blocker or calcium-channel blocker may be used if the symptoms are less severe. If the heart rate is high, it may be necessary to terminate the arrhythmia by the use of a temporary pacing wire (Lazar and Parwani, 2006).

Atrial fibrillation

Atrial fibrillation (often referred to as AF) is a very common arrhythmia. It occurs when there are many foci in the atria all firing through re-entry circuits, in a chaotic fashion. As a result, the atria lose their kick and cardiac output can be reduced by up to 25% (Jevon and Ewens, 2007). There is no electrical synchronisation within the atria and therefore no P waves are present. The foci in the atria may fire at up to 600 times each minute and thus they *quiver* instead of contracting. Instead of P waves, there are *f waves*, which show as an erratic baseline waveform. The rate is very irregular and may be very rapid.

CAUSES OF ATRIAL FIBRILLATION

Smoking

Caffeine

Alcohol

Anxiety and stress

Hypoxia

Hypotension

Electrolyte disturbances

Acute myocardial infarction

Pulmonary embolism

Chronic obstructive pulmonary disease

Atrial fibrillation can be a sustained arrhythmia or can occur paroxysmally. The ventricular rate can vary. It depends how many of the impulses pass through the AV node to stimulate ventricular contraction. The QRS complexes are described as irregularly irregular and T waves are unidentifiable.

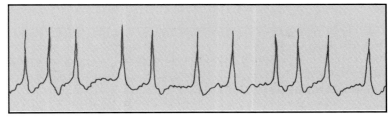

Fig. 3.7 *Atrial fibrillation*

Management

If the patient is unstable and the arrhythmia has been present for less than 48 hours, the treatment of choice is electrical cardioversion (see Chapter 5) (National Institute for Health and Clinical Excellence, 2006; Lazar and Clark, 2007). If the ventricular rate is very rapid, carotid sinus massage (Fig. 3.9) may be useful for slowing the heart rate (Levine *et al.*, 2008).

If cardioversion does not convert the heart back to sinus rhythm, or if AF is persistent, the decision to perform pharmacologic conversion may be made. In this case, an intravenous antiarrhythmic agent will be used. In the absence of structural heart disease (coronary artery disease or left ventricular dysfunction), a class Ic drug (see page 83) such as flecainide or propafenone is used. In the presence of structural heart disease, amiodarone should be the drug of choice (National Institute for Health and Clinical Excellence, 2006).

Anticoagulation is also necessary. This is because when the atria are fibrillating they do not empty correctly so there is an increased chance of clot formation (National Institute for Health and Clinical Excellence, 2006).

Atrial tachycardia

Atrial tachycardia is often referred to as supraventricular tachycardia (SVT). It is indeed a type of supraventricular tachycardia but so are all types of tachycardia that originate *above* the ventricles (i.e. they are *supra*ventricular).

Atrial tachycardia is caused by an abnormal focus in the atria which fires at a rate in excess of 150 b.p.m. (and can reach 250 b.p.m.). It is often associated with stress and/or stimulants but usually manifests in digoxin toxicity and primary or secondary heart conditions and it can lead to more serious arrhythmias.

P waves are often superimposed on the T waves of the preceding beats and thus the T wave may appear distorted. The P waves are usually followed by a normal QRS complex.

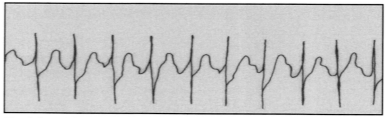

Fig. 3.8 *Atrial tachycardia*

The rhythm is often regular but it may be irregular if there is an AV block present and it can occur as paroxysmal atrial tachycardia. Multifocal atrial tachycardia (MAT) occurs when there are several foci that intermittently fire.

Management

If there is no underlying cause, the tachycardia is transient and the patient is asymptomatic, no treatment is necessary – but the patient should be observed. However, with a sustained atrial tachycardia, even if the patient is asymptomatic, the cause should be determined and treated.

CAUSES OF ATRIAL TACHYCARDIA

Smoking

Caffeine

Stress

Primary or secondary cardiac disease

Digoxin toxicity (most common cause)

Sustained atrial tachycardia, as with sinus tachycardia, can severely reduce cardiac output because of the reduction in ventricular filling time (so there is less blood in the ventricles to pump into the circulation). In addition to this, the heart is working harder in an attempt to maintain the circulation and therefore needs more oxygen, which it cannot get because of the reduction in cardiac output – this chain of events can lead to heart failure. Symptoms of reduced cardiac output are produced and treatment should be instigated to slow the heart rate and increase the power of ventricular contraction. Depending on how unstable the patient is as a result of the arrhythmia, the condition is treated with adenosine or amiodarone or electrical cardioversion (Jevon and Ewens, 2007). Carotid sinus massage can sometimes be successful in slowing the heart rate in the first instance.

Carotid sinus massage can be used either to diagnose or to treat atrial tachycardia but it is to be avoided in older patients (Levine *et al.*, 2008). When the carotid sinus is massaged, the vagus nerve is stimulated and therefore the firing of the SA node is inhibited, slowing the heart rate down. However, a number of complications are associated with carotid sinus massage – bradycardia, asystole, reduced blood pressure as a result of vasodilation, ventricular arrhythmias and cerebral vascular accident. Therefore, it should only be carried out by experienced healthcare professionals when resuscitation equipment is to hand.

Carotid sinus massage is illustrated in Fig. 3.9.

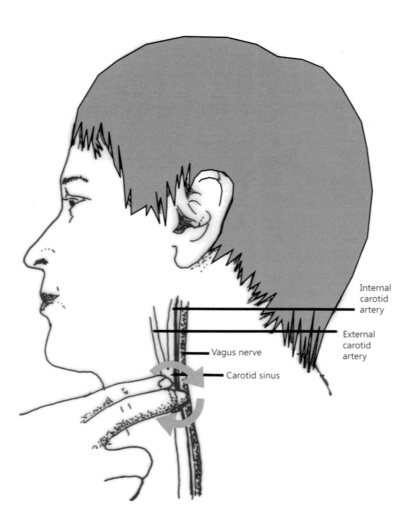

Internal carotid artery

External carotid artery

Vagus nerve

Carotid sinus

Fig. 3.9 *Carotid sinus massage*

ARRHYTHMIAS ARISING AT THE ATRIOVENTRICULAR JUNCTION (including AV blocks)

In critical and acute care areas, the most common arrhythmias seen (that arise at the AV junction, i.e. around the area of the AV node and bundle of His) are **junctional escape rhythm** and **AV block**.

Junctional escape rhythms

If the SA node fails to initiate impulses and another focus within the atria does not take over as pacemaker, the AV node may take over. This causes abnormal conduction as the impulse spreads *upwards* over the atria (instead of downwards). The rate is slower than normal because, as mentioned previously, the lower down the conducting system the impulses are generated, the slower the rate will be.

When monitoring in lead II, a junctional escape rhythm can be determined by a rate of 60 b.p.m. or less, with inverted P waves. The P waves may be inverted because the positive deflection denotes the downward wave of depolarisation; as the impulse originates in the AV node the wave of depolarisation passes in an *upward* direction over the atria and will therefore be seen as a *negative* deflection on the ECG.

However, P waves may be absent if atrial and ventricular depolarisation occurs simultaneously because the P wave will be hidden within the more powerful QRS complex.

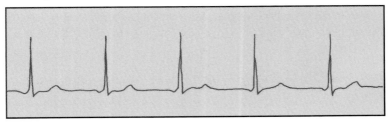

Fig. 3.10 *Junctional escape rhythm*

It is possible to see inverted P waves when the rhythm arises low in the atria; inverted P waves do not automatically demonstrate nodal rhythm.

You can determine this by considering the PR interval. If the PR interval is less than 0.12 seconds long, it is nodal rhythm, but if there is a normal PR interval, the rhythm originated in the atria and you are looking at something other than junctional escape rhythm.

CAUSES OF JUNCTIONAL ESCAPE RHYTHMS

Hypoxia

Digoxin toxicity

Cardiac disease

Sick sinus syndrome

Myocardial infarction

Cardiac surgery

Drugs that may cause bradycardia

Complete heart block

Management

If the patient is asymptomatic, generally the arrhythmia itself is not treated but, if necessary, the underlying cause is. Junctional escape rhythm, as the name suggests, serves as an 'escape' mechanism to maintain the heart rate during periods of bradycardia or asystole and it should not be suppressed (Beinart *et al.*, 2006). In patients with complete heart block, or symptomatic sick sinus syndrome, a permanent pacemaker may be needed. An anticholinergic agent such as atropine may be required if symptomatic bradycardia is present.

N.B. An accelerated junctional escape rhythm will result in tachycardia.

First-degree AV block

First-degree AV (or heart) block is generally not dangerous in itself and the arrhythmia is not treated as it does not usually affect cardiac output.

At first glance it will appear to be normal sinus rhythm, but on closer examination, it is recognised by an extended PR interval of greater than 0.2 seconds (five small squares on the EGG paper) (Docherty and Douglas, 2003). This means there is a delay at the atrioventricular junction before the impulse passes into the bundle of His. The P wave will be followed by a normal QRS complex and T wave and the rate will not be affected.

First-degree AV block may occur normally in a healthy patient.

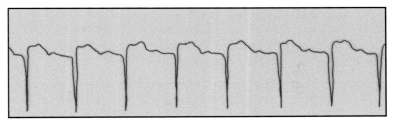

Fig. 3.11 *First-degree AV block*

Management

If the patient is asymptomatic, the arrhythmia is not treated. However, a delay in conduction means there is a problem in the conducting system and therefore should be monitored.

The underlying cause should be treated, if necessary, because first-degree block can progress to more serious forms of heart block.

CAUSES OF FIRST-DEGREE AV BLOCK

(*May occur normally in a healthy patient*)

Myocardial infarction

Degenerative cardiac disease

Most commonly caused by drugs that depress
AV conduction: (e.g. beta-blockers, digoxin,
calcium-channel blockers)

Second-degree AV block

There are two types of second-degree heart block known as **Mobitz type I** and **Mobitz type II**. Mobitz type I is also commonly known as **Wenckebach** phenomenon (because it was discovered by a man called Wenckebach).

Mobitz type I (Wenckebach phenomenon)

This is a cyclical rhythm recognised by a progressively increasing PR interval. It continues to increase until eventually the impulse is blocked and cannot stimulate ventricular depolarisation so the next QRS complex is dropped. The sequence then begins again.

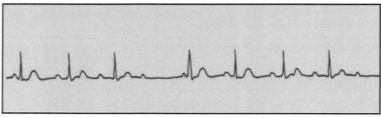

Fig. 3.12 *Mobitz type I second-degree AV block*

Management

If the patient is asymptomatic, the arrhythmia is not treated as it is usually transient. However, as with first-degree AV block, a delay in conduction means there is a problem in the conducting system and this should therefore be monitored.

> **CAUSES OF SECOND-DEGREE AV BLOCK (MOBITZ TYPE I)**
>
> Myocardial infarction
>
> Degenerative cardiac disease
>
> Drugs that depress AV conduction (most commonly) such as beta-blockers, digoxin and calcium-channel blockers

The underlying cause should be treated, if necessary, because Mobitz type I block can progress to more serious forms of heart block. If the rhythm is prolonged and causes a reduction in cardiac output, it may be necessary to give atropine. A temporary transvenous pacing wire may be required to support the patient until the arrhythmia has resolved.

Mobitz type II

A Mobitz type II second-degree AV block is more serious than a type I block but is less common. This arrhythmia usually requires intervention because it frequently progresses to high-grade block or complete heart block. It is easily recognised as frequent impulses fail to pass through the AV node and are seen as missed beats (no QRS complex) or it takes two P waves to stimulate a QRS complex. This is known as a 2:1 block, meaning every other QRS complex is dropped.

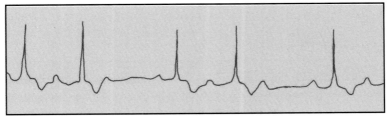

Fig. 3.13 *Mobitz type II second-degree AV block*

A high-grade AV block exists if there is a 3:1 or higher ratio of P waves to QRS complexes. This will result in a drastic reduction in cardiac output and rapidly progresses to complete heart block.

CAUSES OF SECOND-DEGREE AV BLOCK (MOBITZ TYPE II)

Myocardial infarction

Degenerative heart disease

Digoxin toxicity

Management

Transcutaneous pacing or a temporary transvenous pacing wire is indicated for all patients with Mobitz type II block, including asymptomatic patients, as patients with Mobitz II second-degree AV block usually progress to complete heart block (Levine and Brown, 2006). An anticholinergic drug such as atropine may also be required.

Third-degree AV block

Third-degree heart block, also known as **complete heart block,** is potentially life-threatening and requires immediate intervention. The atria depolarise normally but the impulse cannot pass through the AV node, so no impulses are passed from the atria to the ventricles (Docherty and Douglas, 2003).

A focus in the ventricles may take over but the ventricles beat at a slower rate than the atria and the atria and ventricles depolarise and contract independently of one another.

A focus in the His–Purkinje system may take over as the pacemaker, causing ventricular depolarisation. The ventricular rate will be slow and the patient will immediately suffer symptoms of a reduced cardiac output.

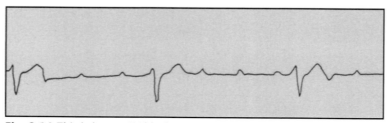

Fig. 3.14 *Third-degree AV block*

Therefore a normal and regular atrial rate will be seen, usually with normal P waves which do not relate to the QRS complexes. P waves can sometimes be disguised by a QRS complex or T wave. The ventricular rate is also regular but much slower than the atrial rate and the QRS complexes are usually widened because they are initiated lower down the conducting system than normal. If a ventricular focus does not take over as pacemaker, ventricular 'standstill' will follow which is seen as a row of P waves with no QRS complexes.

CAUSES OF THIRD-DEGREE AV BLOCK

Myocardial infarction

Degenerative cardiac disease

Digoxin toxicity

Drugs that depress AV conduction (beta-blockers and calcium-channel blockers)

Management

In a critically ill patient, this arrhythmia will usually drastically reduce cardiac output. It is a medical emergency and it requires immediate drug therapy in order to improve the ventricular rate.

Atropine is usually given and inotropic agents may be required to support the patient's circulation. The insertion of a temporary transvenous pacing wire is often necessary until the cause of the block has been resolved.

If the block is permanent, a permanent pacemaker will subsequently be required (Hand, 2002).

VENTRICULAR ARRHYTHMIAS

Ventricular extrasystoles

Ventricular extrasystoles, also known as ventricular ectopic beats or premature ventricular contractions (PVCs), arise from an irritable focus within the ventricles, firing randomly. They are very common and can occur quite naturally in healthy patients. They do not necessarily cause any symptoms or problems.

They are easily recognised as they have wide and bizarre QRS complexes which are therefore easy to diagnose. During a ventricular extrasystole, there is a reduced (or no) cardiac output and if they don't occur frequently, they are usually of no importance and are left untreated. However, if they are very frequent or occur in salvos (i.e. two or more together), or occur in a repeating pattern (such as in bigeminy or trigeminy), or occur in a patient with cardiac disease or problems, then they can cause a reduction in cardiac output or lead to more serious ventricular arrhythmias, in which case treatment will be necessary.

There are various types of ventricular extrasystoles that result in various arrhythmias.

CAUSES OF VENTRICULAR EXTRASYSTOLES

Use of substances such as alcohol, caffeine, tobacco and cocaine

Electrolyte imbalance

Hypoxia

Hypothermia

Myocardial infarction

Metabolic acidosis

Digoxin toxicity

Unifocal ventricular extrasystoles

Unifocal ventricular extrasystoles are all the same shape and size and are caused by an irritable ectopic focus in the ventricles firing before it should. Conduction through the myocardium is abnormal and ventricular depolarisation is delayed, resulting in a wide QRS complex.

Occurring infrequently, these arrhythmias are of little or no consequence but if there is a salvo of three or more then this is – by definition – ventricular tachycardia (Hand, 2002) and this indicates an irritable or unstable myocardium.

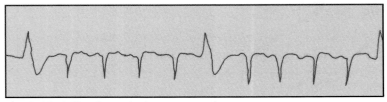

Fig. 3.15 *Unifocal ventricular extrasystoles*

Multifocal ventricular extrasystoles

Multifocal ventricular extrasystoles are more dangerous than unifocal ventricular extrasystoles because there is more than one irritable focus in the ventricular muscle. They can be easily recognised by their differing shapes and sizes. These arrhythmias can lead to more serious arrhythmias, or even lethal arrhythmias such as ventricular fibrillation.

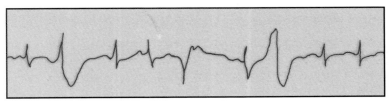

Fig. 3.16 *Multifocal ventricular extrasystoles*

Bigeminy

Bigeminy is caused by an abnormal focus in the ventricular muscle and is recognised by a unifocal ventricular ectopic beat after each normal sinus beat. If this is prolonged, it causes reduced cardiac output and hypotension and will require intervention.

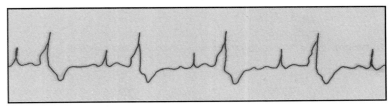

Fig. 3.17 *Bigeminy*

Trigeminy

Trigeminy is recognised by a unifocal ventricular extrasystole after every two sinus beats, following a regular pattern. As with bigeminy, if this is prolonged it will cause reduced cardiac output and hypotension and will require intervention.

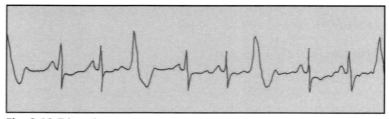

Fig. 3.18 *Trigeminy*

R-on-T phenomenon

R-on-T phenomenon occurs when a ventricular extrasystole occurs at the peak of the T wave of the preceding beat (i.e. during ventricular repolarisation, when the heart is resting). This is very dangerous and can lead to ventricular tachycardia or ventricular fibrillation.

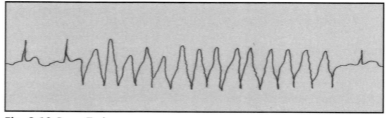

Fig. 3.19 *R-on-T phenomenon*

Management of ventricular extrasystoles and related rhythms

If ventricular extrasystoles are infrequent and the patient is asymptomatic, no treatment is necessary. However, if they are frequent and/or produce symptoms of reduced cardiac output, treatment will need to be instigated.

The treatment depends upon the cause of the problem. For example:

- If caused by **hypoxia**, oxygen administration is required or the oxygen concentration should be increased.
- If caused by **acidosis**, correct the acidosis.
- If caused by **hypokalaemia** (low potassium), **hypocalcaemia** (low calcium) or **hypomagnesaemia** (low magnesium), give intravenous supplementation.

N.B. If they are frequent and/or dangerous, give antiarrhythmic drugs.

However, remember that antiarrhythmic agents may worsen existing arrhythmias or cause new rhythm disturbances; this is known as the proarrhythmic effect (Marini and Wheeler, 2006). Intravenous amiodarone is used for the acute treatment of ventricular extrasystoles, and beta-blockers and calcium-channel blockers may also be used (Marini and Wheeler, 2006).

Ventricular tachycardia

Ventricular tachycardia (VT), also known as broad complex tachycardia, is present if a focus in the ventricular muscle fires at high frequency and more than three ventricular ectopic beats occur in a row at a rate of 100–250 b.p.m. In effect it causes rapidly repeated ventricular extrasystoles.

There are no P waves present, the QRS complexes are wide and slightly irregular and may vary slightly in shape. It may occur paroxysmally and cause no symptoms, but sustained VT is very dangerous and is usually a life-threatening arrhythmia that often precedes ventricular fibrillation. Therefore it requires immediate intervention.

VT can be *monomorphic* or *polymorphic* and either can be pulseless.

Monomorphic ventricular tachycardia

Monomorphic VT is caused by a single ectopic focus firing rapidly and all the complexes look the same (Fig. 3.20).

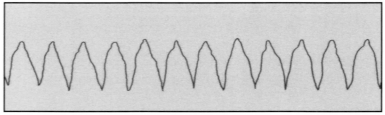

Fig. 3.20 *Monomorphic ventricular tachycardia*

Polymorphic ventricular tachycardia

Polymorphic VT occurs when there are more than one ectopic foci firing and the complexes therefore change in shape and size (Docherty and Douglas, 2003) (Fig. 3.21). An example of this is torsades de pointes, which may be paroxysmal and is often caused by drugs.

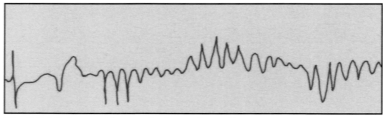

Fig. 3.21 *Polymorphic ventricular tachycardia*

When VT is sustained, the patient often becomes pulseless and will collapse as a result because ventricular filling time is severely reduced, as is the force of contraction. Therefore, cardiac output is reduced and, consequently, so is the blood pressure. The condition may degenerate into ventricular fibrillation, causing immediate cardiac arrest (Hand, 2002). Immediate action is therefore necessary.

Management

The management of patients with VT depends on the symptoms produced.

If the patient is **pulseless**, it is treated in the same way as ventricular fibrillation, namely by defibrillation and cardiopulmonary resuscitation (following the UK Resuscitation Council's algorithm).

If the **pulse is present** but the patient is unstable, DC synchronised cardioversion is needed immediately (Levine *et al.*, 2008).

A stable patient will be treated with amiodarone and the cause corrected. If amiodarone is ineffective, DC synchronised cardioversion will be needed (Levine *et al.*, 2008).

CAUSES OF VENTRICULAR TACHYCARDIA

Myocardial infarction

Proarrhythmic effects of some antiarrhythmic agents

Electrolyte imbalance

Heart failure

Valvular disease

Ventricular fibrillation

Ventricular fibrillation (VF) is caused by numerous irritable foci within the myocardium firing rapidly and chaotically. The effect of this is that the ventricles *quiver* rather than contract and thus there is no cardiac output; the physiological effects are the same as asystole. However, there is a greater chance of survival as there is still some electrical activity.

The finer the trace, the less chance there is of survival.

Untreated VF will usually cause sudden death. Rhythm strips of fine and coarse VF are shown overpage.

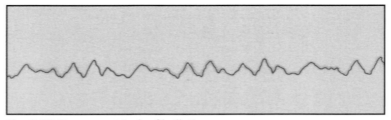

Fig. 3.22 *Coarse ventricular fibrillation*

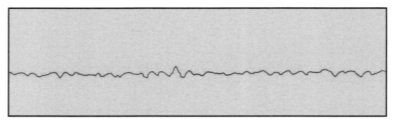

Fig. 3.23 *Fine ventricular fibrillation*

Management

If VF is suspected, immediately check the patient (VF can be mimicked by external electrical interference). If the patient is unresponsive, treatment in the form of defibrillation must be instigated immediately following the UK Resuscitation Council's algorithm, as the patient is in cardiac arrest. If there is any doubt about whether the rhythm is asystole or fine VF (Fig. 3.23) *do not* attempt defibrillation. Instead, continue chest compression and ventilation (Resuscitation Council UK, 2009).

Consider giving a single precordial thump (a sharp blow to the lower third of the sternum) when cardiac arrest is confirmed rapidly after a witnessed and monitored sudden collapse and there is no defibrillator immediately to hand. A precordial thump should be undertaken immediately after confirmation of cardiac arrest but *only* by healthcare professionals trained in the technique (Resuscitation Council UK, 2009). Cardiopulmonary resuscitation must be initiated if defibrillation is delayed for any reason to ensure oxygen delivery. Intravenous epinephrine is administered if defibrillation does not immediately revert the rhythm to sinus rhythm (Resuscitation Council UK, 2009).

CAUSES OF VENTRICULAR FIBRILLATION

Hypoxia

Electrolyte imbalances

Acid–base disturbances

Ventricular tachycardia and other arrhythmias

Digoxin toxicity

Hypothermia

Heart disease

Myocardial infarction

ASYSTOLE

Asystole literally means 'no systole' and therefore there is no electrical activity and no mechanical contraction of the heart (this is ventricular 'standstill').

Without immediate treatment, asystole is rapidly irreversible and death ensues. The ECG trace is seen as a flat line.

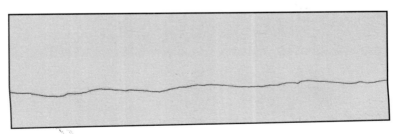

Fig. 3.24 *Asystole*

Management
If asystole is suspected, check the patient immediately. Asystole can be mimicked by something as simple as electrode detachment. Ensure that

fine VF is excluded by turning up the gain on the monitor. If the patient is pulseless and unresponsive, cardiopulmonary resuscitation must be instigated immediately, together with a single dose of intravenous atropine and repeated doses of epinephrine, following the UK Resuscitation Council's algorithm.

It should be noted that treatment for a patient in asystole (particularly sustained asystole) is unlikely to be successful.

CAUSES OF ASYSTOLE

Untreated ventricular fibrillation

Severe hypoxia

Severe electrolyte imbalances

Severe acid–base disturbances

Myocardial infarction

Hypothermia

Consolidation

You will consolidate your learning from this chapter by completing Chapter 5 (but do work through Chapter 4 before you do this!).

Notes

Arrhythmia interventions

Many of the arrhythmias discussed within this workbook require no treatment, because they will not affect cardiac output (e.g. occasional unifocal ventricular extrasystoles). However, many arrhythmias may compromise a patient's cardiovascular system and some of them are even life-threatening. It is important to remember that what may appear to be a benign arrhythmia may lead to a more serious arrhythmia – particularly in a patient who is already critically ill – and this is why the importance of accurate monitoring cannot be stressed enough.

In this chapter we will consider some of the treatment options for the arrhythmias we have considered throughout the book. Appropriate management requires precise diagnosis and appropriate treatment of the underlying cause (British Medical Association and Royal Pharmaceutical Society of Great Britain, 2009).

> **WHEN AN ARRHYTHMIA IS DETECTED**
> Check ABCs (airway, breathing, circulation).
> Commence cardiopulmonary resuscitation without delay (if necessary).
> If the patient is asymptomatic then often no treatment is required.
> If cardiac output is affected then treatment is necessary.

Treatment is aimed symptomatically and/or causally. Table 4.1 (overpage) summarises appropriate interventions for the different arrhythmias.

Drug and non-drug interventions

The interventions listed in Table 4.1 are instigated if the patient is demonstrating symptoms of reduced cardiac output. Where no symptoms are apparent, or are unlikely, treatment is usually not necessary. Arrhythmias marked with an asterisk (*) require the treatment stated, regardless of the symptoms.

Table 4.1 Specific interventions for arrhythmias

Arrhythmia	Non-drug intervention	Drug intervention
Sinus arrhythmia	Treat cause if symptomatic	Treat cause if symptomatic
Sinus bradycardia	Transcutaneous or transvenous pacing	Atropine
Sinus tachycardia	If caused by haemorrhage, stop bleeding and replace fluid	Beta-blockers Calcium-channel blockers
Premature atrial contractions	Treat cause if symptomatic	Digoxin (if problematic)
Atrial flutter	Direct-current synchronised cardioversion (if tachycardia, use transcutaneous or transvenous pacing)	Beta-blockers Verapamil
Atrial fibrillation	Direct-current synchronised cardioversion (if less than 48 hours from onset of arrhythmia) Carotid sinus massage	Flecainide or propafenone (if no structural heart disease) Amiodarone (if structural heart disease) Anticoagulant drugs
Atrial tachycardia	Carotid sinus massage Direct-current synchronised cardioversion	Adenosine Amiodarone
Junctional escape rhythm	Treat cause if symptomatic	Atropine (if arrhythmia causes symptomatic bradycardia)
First-degree AV block	Treat underlying cause	Treat underlying cause
Mobitz type I second-degree heart block	Transcutaneous pacing Transvenous pacing	Atropine

Table 4.1 (*cont.*)

Arrhythmia	Non-drug intervention	Drug intervention
Mobitz type II second-degree heart block*	Transcutaneous pacing Transvenous pacing	Atropine
Third-degree AV block*	Transcutaneous or transvenous pacing (if arrhythmia is permanent, permanent pacemaker is required)	Atropine
Unifocal ventricular extrasystoles	Treat underlying cause	Amiodarone Beta-blockers Calcium-channel blockers Lidocaine
Multifocal ventricular extrasystoles	Treat underlying cause	Amiodarone Beta-blockers Calcium-channel blockers Lidocaine
Bigiminy	Treat underlying cause	Amiodarone Beta-blockers Calcium-channel blockers Lidocaine
Trigeminy	Treat underlying cause	Amiodarone Beta-blockers Calcium-channel blockers Lidocaine
R-on-T phenomenon*	Treat underlying cause	Amiodarone Beta-blockers Calcium-channel blockers Lidocaine
Monomorphic ventricular tachycardia*	**If pulseless:** defibrillation and/or cardiopulmonary resuscitation **If pulse present:** (patient unstable) DC synchronised cardioversion; (patient stable, amiodarone ineffective) DC synchronised cardioversion	Epinephrine Amiodarone
Polymorphic ventricular tachycardia*	**If pulseless:** defibrillation and/or cardiopulmonary resuscitation **If pulse present:** (patient unstable) DC synchronised cardioversion; (patient stable, amiodarone ineffective) DC synchronised cardioversion	Epinephrine Amiodarone

Table 4.1 (*cont.*)

Arrhythmia	Non-drug intervention	Drug intervention
Ventricular fibrillation*	Defibrillation and/or cardiopulmonary resuscitation	Epinephrine
Asystole*	Cardiopulmonary resuscitation	Epinephrine Atropine

*Require treatment regardless of symptoms.

Drugs used for arrhythmia treatment

Table 4.2 lists the drugs used for arrhythmia treatment, according to the Vaughan-Williams classification of antiarrhythmic drugs (Anaesthesia UK, 2008; British Medical Association and Royal Pharmaceutical Society of Great Britain, 2009).

Table 4.2 Drugs used for arrhythmia treatment (Anaesthesia UK, 2008; British Medical Association and Royal Pharmaceutical Society of Great Britain, 2009)

Class	Mechanism	Drug(s)	Uses
I	Sodium-channel blockers that *prolong* the action potential	Quinidine Procainamide Disopyramide	Supraventricular arrhythmias
Ib	Sodium-channel blockers that *shorten* the action potential	Lidocaine	Ventricular extrasystoles
Ic	Sodium-channel blockers that *don't affect* action potential	Flecainide Propafenone	Ventricular extrasystoles
II	Beta-blockers	Atenolol Esmolol Propanalol	Sinus tachycardia Atrial fibrillation Atrial tachycardia Ventricular extrasystoles
III	Potassium-channel blockers	Amiodarone	Atrial fibrillation Ventricular extrasystoles Stable ventricular tachycardia

Table 4.2 (*cont.*)

Class	Mechanism	Drug(s)	Uses
IV	Calcium-channel blockers	Verapamil Diltiazem	Sinus tachycardia Atrial flutter Atrial fibrillation Atrial tachycardia Ventricular extrasystoles
V	Other mechanisms	Digoxin	Premature atrial contractions Atrial fibrillation Atrial tachycardia
		Atropine	Sinus bradycardia Junctional escape rhythm Second-degree heart block (Mobitz I and II) Third-degree heart block Asystole
		Epinephrine	Ventricular fibrillation Asystole

Defibrillation

The delivery of a direct electrical current through the heart depolarises the myocardium allowing the sinoatrial node to resume its normal pacemaker function (Levine *et al.*, 2008).

Automatic external defibrillators

An automatic external defibrillator (AED) should be used wherever possible. All healthcare professionals should consider the use of an AED to be an integral component of basic life support (Resuscitation Council UK, 2009). They are described as sophisticated, reliable, safe, computerised devices that deliver defibrillatory shocks to victims of cardiac arrest by giving visual and voice prompts to rescuers (Resuscitation Council UK, 2009).

Manual defibrillator

Where a manual defibrillator is in use, wherever possible, apply self-adhesive defibrillator pads, attached to the defibrillator through an interface cable, rather than paddles because this will reduce the risk of sparks and the operator will not have to lean over the patient (Resuscitation Council UK, 2009).

Defibrillator paddles

When using defibrillator paddles, water-based gel pads should be placed between the paddles and the patient's skin. The paddles should be placed in the appropriate position:

- The right (sternal) electrode is placed below the clavicle to the right of the sternum.
- The apical paddle is placed vertically in the mid-axillary line, level with the V6 ECG electrode's position (Resuscitation Council UK, 2009).

The paddles should be pressed firmly to the chest wall with an optimal force of 8 kg (Resuscitation Council UK, 2009). A shock of between 150–360 Joules is delivered when the patient is in ventricular fibrillation.

Safety considerations

Turn off oxygen supplementation or remove the oxygen mask or nasal cannulae and move them at least 1 metre away before the shock is delivered. Sparks from poorly applied paddles may cause a fire in an oxygen-rich environment (Resuscitation Council UK, 2009). Remove any transdermal drug patches before a shock is delivered (Resuscitation Council UK, 2009). This is particularly important for GTN (glyceryl trinitrate) patches because they may explode.

> **Whenever defibrillation is carried out,
> the UK Resuscitation Council's guidelines
> and algorithms should be followed.**
>
> **Defibrillation should *only* be carried out by trained
> healthcare professionals.**

Cardioversion

Cardioversion is carried out in the same manner as defibrillation but the direct-current (DC) shock is delivered in synchrony with the peak of the R wave. The defibrillator has a 'synchronise' switch which is utilised for cardioversion. The other major differences are that the conscious patient will usually require sedation, and the intensity of the shock is usually less.

Approaches to energy selection

There are two approaches to energy selection for cardioversion. Some physicians feel that it is best to select the highest possible energy in order to maximise the chance of initial success, to minimise the number of shocks, and to lessen the exposure to sedative agents. Other physicians prefer to follow an 'escalating energy' protocol. This method also allows cardioversion at the lowest energy for each individual patient and may prevent high cumulative doses in some (Adgey, 2005). Current evidence suggests that the majority of patients will be successfully cardioverted by shocks of 200 Joules, and it appears that only a very small percentage of patients benefit from stronger shocks (Adgey, 2005). Note that antero-posterior electrode placement may be more effective than the traditional antero-apical position in cardioversion of atrial fibrillation, although either position is acceptable (Resuscitation Council UK, 2009).

Pacing

Temporary pacing

A pacemaker is a device that generates an electrical impulse from a pulse generator, which is then transmitted through the heart causing depolarisation. This in turn brings about contraction of the myocardium. Temporary pacemakers are used in emergency and acute situations until the arrhythmia has resolved or until a permanent pacemaker can be fitted if necessary.

Transcutaneous pacing

Transcutaneous pacing is used in an emergency situation and is a simple, non-invasive process of applying external electrodes to the anterior chest wall, or on the patient's anterior chest wall and one on the patient's back. Electrical impulses are generated and these pass through the skin to the myocardium and thus pace the heart. Transvenous pacing is often subsequently required.

Transvenous pacing

Transvenous pacing is used in emergency and acute situations. A pacing wire is passed into the right atrium or ventricle via the internal jugular or subclavian vein and attached to a pulse generator.

Electrical impulses are generated that pass through the wire and stimulate the myocardium, causing it to depolarise and contract (Fig. 4.1).

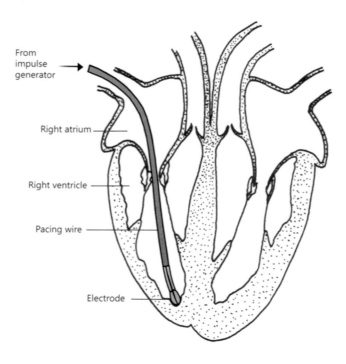

Fig. 4.1 *Transvenous pacing wire in situ*

When a patient has a pacemaker in situ, a **pacing spike** is seen on the ECG trace because the ECG will pick up the electrical impulse generated by the pacemaker (see Fig. 4.2).

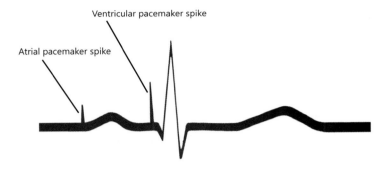

Fig. 4.2 *Pacing spike*

Now check how much you have learnt in this chapter by completing the *Consolidation* section overpage.

Consolidation

See pages 144–145 for answers

4.1   Fill in the table below as completely as possible.

Arrhythmia	Symptoms	Non-drug intervention	Drug intervention
Sinus arrhythmia			
Sinus bradycardia			
Sinus tachycardia			
Premature atrial contractions			
Atrial flutter			
Atrial fibrillation			
Atrial tachycardia			
Junctional escape rhythm			
First-degree AV block			
Mobitz type I second-degree heart block			

Arrhythmia	Symptoms	Non-drug intervention	Drug intervention
Mobitz type II second-degree heart block*			
Third-degree AV block*			
Unifocal ventricular extrasystoles			
Multifocal ventricular extrasystoles			
Bigeminy			
Trigeminy			
R-on-T phenomenon			
Monomorphic ventricular tachycardia			
Polymorphic ventricular tachycardia			
Ventricular fibrillation			
Asystole			

4.2   Fill in as much detail as possible on the following table.

Class	Mechanism	Drug(s)	Uses
IA			
IB			
IC			
II			
III			
IV			
V			

4.3   How does defibrillation work?

_____

_____

4.4   What is an AED?

_____

_____

4.5   What are the advantages of using self-adhesive defibrillator pads?

_____

_____

4.6   When using a manual defibrillator, in what positions are defibrillator paddles placed?

_____

_____

4.7   What is the optimal force that should be applied to defibrillator paddles?

_____

4.8   When a patient is in ventricular fibrillation, what is the intensity of the DC shock that is delivered?

_____

4.9   What are the safety considerations when defibrillation is to be carried out?

_____

_____

_____

_____

_____

_____

4.10 What are the major differences between defibrillation and cardioversion?

_____

_____

_____

_____

4.11 How do temporary pacemakers work?

_____

_____

_____

4.12 In what situations are temporary pacemakers used?

_____

_____

4.13 When and how is transcutaneous pacing used?

_____

_____

_____

_____

4.14   When and how is transvenous pacing used?

_____

_____

_____

_____

4.15   What is notable about the ECG trace when a pacemaker is in situ?

_____

Notes

Chapter 5

Putting it all together

Now that we have considered all of the necessary information, we need to put this information to the test. When considering a rhythm strip, it is helpful to approach diagnosis with a systematic evaluation that will help you to determine the rhythm.

The following six steps can by applied systematically to each arrhythmia you deal with.

Step 1—Consider whether the rhythm is life-threatening

If it is life-threatening, summon help and instigate the appropriate algorithm (Resuscitation Council UK, 2008).

Step 2—Consider the heart rate

- **Bradycardia**   Less than 60 b.p.m.
- **Normal rate**   Between 60 and 100 b.p.m.
- **Tachycardia**   More than 100 b.p.m.

Step 3—Consider the P waves

If P waves are present:

- Are they normal in appearance?
- Does one P wave occur before each QRS complex?

Step 4—Consider the PR interval

- Is the PR interval of normal duration (0.12–0.2 seconds)?
- Is the interval prolonged?
- Is the interval shortened?
- Is it consistent?

Step 5—Consider the QRS complex

- Is the QRS complex normal in duration (0.06–0.12 seconds)?
- Is the QRS consistent in duration?
- Are the complexes of normal shape and configuration?
- Is the QRS consistent in form?

Step 6—Consider the RR interval

- Is the RR interval consistent?
- If it is inconsistent, is there some pattern in the variation?

Now, bearing these six steps in mind, see if you can work out what arrhythmias are shown in the ECG strips on the following pages and answer the specific questions about each one.

Answers are given on pages 146–152.

5.1 What is this rhythm?

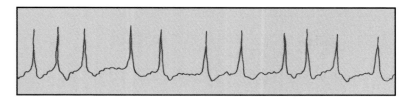

5.2 What action would you take if a patient was demonstrating this rhythm?

5.3 What is this rhythm?

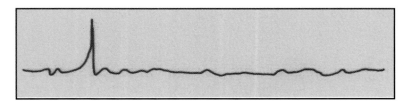

5.4 What action would you take if a patient was demonstrating this rhythm?

5.5 What is this rhythm?

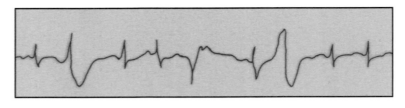

5.6 What action would you take if a patient was demonstrating this rhythm?

_____

_____

_____

5.7 What is this rhythm?

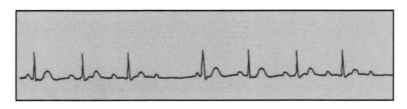

5.8 What action would you take if a patient was demonstrating this rhythm?

_____

_____

_____

5.9 What is this rhythm?

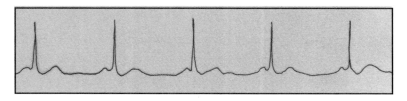

5.10 What action would you take if a patient was demonstrating this rhythm?

_____

_____

_____

5.11 What is this rhythm?

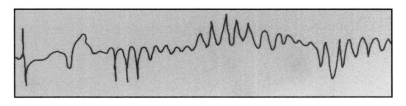

5.12 What action would you take if a patient was demonstrating this rhythm?

_____

_____

_____

5.13 What is this rhythm?

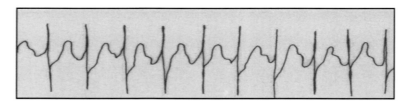

5.14 What action would you take if a patient was demonstrating this rhythm?

_____

_____

_____

5.15 What is this rhythm?

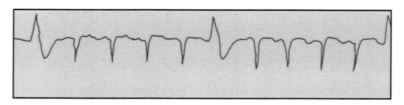

5.16 What action would you take if a patient was demonstrating this rhythm?

_____

_____

_____

5.17 What is this rhythm?

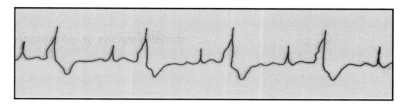

5.18 What action would you take if a patient was demonstrating this rhythm?

_____

_____

_____

5.19 What is this rhythm?

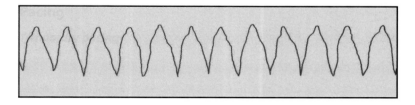

5.20 What action would you take if a patient was demonstrating this rhythm?

_____

_____

_____

5.21 What is this rhythm?

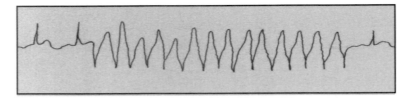

5.22 What action would you take if a patient was demonstrating this rhythm?

_____

_____

_____

5.23 What is this rhythm?

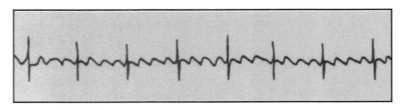

5.24 What action would you take if a patient was demonstrating this rhythm?

_____

_____

_____

5.25 What is this rhythm?

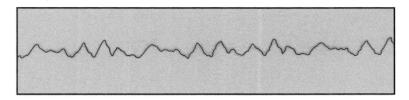

5.26 What action would you take if a patient was demonstrating this rhythm?

_____

_____

_____

5.27 What is this rhythm?

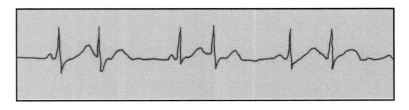

5.28 What action would you take if a patient was demonstrating this rhythm?

_____

_____

_____

5.29 What is this rhythm?

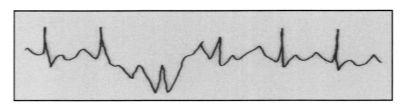

5.30 What action would you take if a patient was demonstrating this rhythm?

_____

_____

_____

5.31 What is this rhythm?

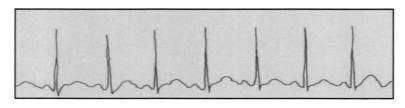

5.32 What action would you take if a patient was demonstrating this rhythm?

_____

_____

_____

5.33 What is this rhythm?

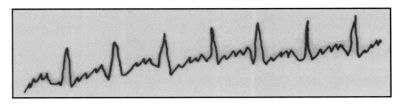

5.34 What action would you take if a patient was demonstrating this rhythm?

_____

_____

_____

5.35 What is this rhythm?

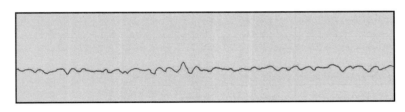

5.36 What action would you take if a patient was demonstrating this rhythm?

_____

_____

_____

5.37 What is this rhythm?

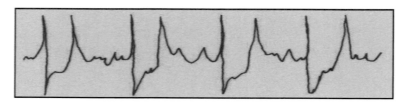

5.38 What action would you take if a patient was demonstrating this rhythm?

_____

_____

_____

5.39 What is this rhythm?

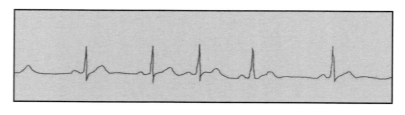

5.40 What action would you take if a patient was demonstrating this rhythm?

_____

_____

_____

5.41 What is this rhythm?

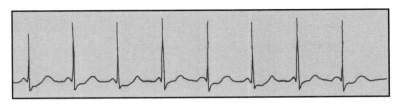

5.42 What action would you take if a patient was demonstrating this rhythm?

_____

_____

_____

5.43 What is this rhythm?

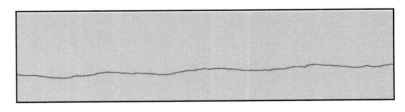

5.44 What action would you take if a patient was demonstrating this rhythm?

_____

_____

_____

5.45 What is this rhythm?

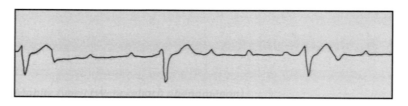

5.46 What action would you take if a patient was demonstrating this rhythm?

_____

_____

_____

5.47 What is this rhythm?

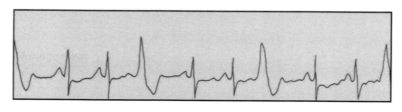

5.48 What action would you take if a patient was demonstrating this rhythm?

_____

_____

_____

5.49 What is this rhythm?

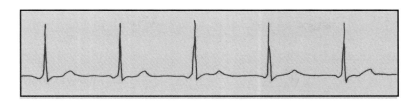

5.50 What action would you take if a patient was demonstrating this rhythm?

_____

_____

_____

5.51 What is this rhythm?

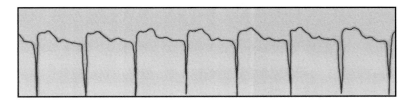

5.52 What action would you take if a patient was demonstrating this rhythm?

_____

_____

_____

5.53 What is this rhythm?

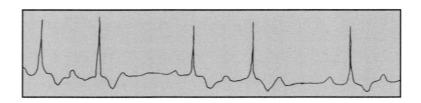

5.54 What action would you take if a patient was demonstrating this rhythm?

_____

_____

_____

5.55 Collect six consecutive cardiac rhythm strips from a patient who is receiving treatment for a problematic arrhythmia and place them on the following pages. For each sample, give an overview of the arrhythmia, state what action was taken and whether this worked or not. Discuss your findings with your mentor.

Sample 1

Place your rhythm strip here.

Give an overview of this arrhythmia.

_____

_____

_____

_____

What action was undertaken?

_____

_____

_____

_____

_____

_____

_____

What effect did the action have?

_____

_____

_____

_____

_____

_____

Sample 2

Place your rhythm strip here.

Give an overview of this arrhythmia.

_____

_____

_____

_____

_____

_____

What action was undertaken?

_____

_____

_____

_____

_____

_____

_____

What effect did the action have?

_____

_____

_____

_____

_____

_____

Sample 3

Place your rhythm strip here.

Give an overview of this arrhythmia.

_____

_____

_____

_____

_____

_____

What action was undertaken?

_____

_____

_____

_____

_____

_____

_____

What effect did the action have?

_____

_____

_____

_____

_____

_____

Sample 4

Place your rhythm strip here.

Give an overview of this arrhythmia.

What action was undertaken?

_____

_____

_____

_____

_____

_____

What effect did the action have?

_____

_____

_____

_____

_____

_____

Sample 5

Place your rhythm strip here.

Give an overview of this arrhythmia.

_____

_____

_____

_____

_____

_____

What action was undertaken?

_____

_____

_____

_____

_____

_____

_____

What effect did the action have?

_____

_____

_____

_____

_____

_____

Sample 6

Place your rhythm strip here.

Give an overview of this arrhythmia.

_____

_____

_____

_____

_____

_____

What action was undertaken?

_____

_____

_____

_____

_____

_____

_____

What effect did the action have?

_____

_____

_____

_____

_____

_____

5.56 Collect six samples from different patients who are experiencing arrhythmias and provide the same information as with the previous samples. Discuss your findings with your mentor.

Sample 1

Place your rhythm strip here.

Give an overview of this arrhythmia.

_____

_____

_____

_____

What action was undertaken?

_____

_____

_____

_____

_____

_____

What effect did the action have?

_____

_____

_____

_____

_____

_____

Sample 2

Place your rhythm strip here.

Give an overview of this arrhythmia.

_____

_____

_____

_____

_____

_____

What action was undertaken?

_____

_____

_____

_____

_____

_____

What effect did the action have?

_____

_____

_____

_____

_____

_____

Sample 3

Place your rhythm strip here.

Give an overview of this arrhythmia.

What action was undertaken?

_____

_____

_____

_____

_____

_____

_____

What effect did the action have?

_____

_____

_____

_____

_____

_____

Sample 4

Place your rhythm strip here.

Give an overview of this arrhythmia.

_____

_____

_____

_____

_____

_____

What action was undertaken?

_____

_____

_____

_____

_____

_____

What effect did the action have?

_____

_____

_____

_____

_____

Sample 5

Place your rhythm strip here.

Give an overview of this arrhythmia.

_____

_____

_____

_____

_____

_____

What action was undertaken?

_____

_____

_____

_____

_____

_____

What effect did the action have?

_____

_____

_____

_____

_____

_____

Sample 6

Place your rhythm strip here.

Give an overview of this arrhythmia.

_____

_____

_____

_____

_____

_____

What action was undertaken?

_____

_____

_____

_____

_____

_____

_____

What effect did the action have?

_____

_____

_____

_____

_____

_____

Sample 6

Place your rhythm strip here.

Give an overview of this arrhythmia.

_____

_____

_____

_____

_____

_____

What action was undertaken?

_____

_____

_____

_____

_____

_____

What effect did the action have?

_____

_____

_____

_____

_____

_____

Congratulations! You've reached the end of this workbook.

Now you can check your answers to the exercises in this chapter on pages 146–152 to make sure you have understood everything.

Notes

Answers and Teaching Notes

1: Anatomy and physiology of the heart

1.1 To circulate blood around the body and therefore oxygen and nutrients to the tissues.

1.2 The heart is a four-chambered double-pump, with the two atria receiving returning blood and directing it to the two ventricles.

1.3 Compare your labels to those on Fig. 1.4 (page 5).

1.4 The epicardium (outer layer), the myocardium (middle layer made up of cardiac muscle) and the endocardium (inner layer).

1.5 Cardiac muscle fibres are involuntary, striated and branched, arranged in interlacing bundles. Each cell has branches that lie close against to the next cell forming junctions called intercalated discs.

1.6. The tricuspid (or right atrioventricular) valve, the mitral (or left atrioventricular) valve, the pulmonary valve (outflow to the pulmonary artery) and the aortic valve (outflow to the aorta). The aortic and pulmonary valves are often referred to as the semilunar valves.

1.7 The venae cavae return blood from the systemic circulation to the right atrium. It passes from the right atrium into the right ventricle via the tricuspid valve. From the right ventricle it passes into the pulmonary artery via the pulmonary valve, and on to the lungs. It picks up oxygen and releases carbon dioxide in the lungs. The oxygenated blood returns to the left side of the heart via the four pulmonary veins. From the left atrium it passes into the left ventricle via the mitral valve and passes from the left ventricle into the aorta via the aortic valve, to be distributed around the systemic circulation.

1.8 The heart is supplied with arterial blood from the right and left coronary arteries (the first branches from the aorta immediately above the aortic valve). These arteries take 4% of the cardiac output from the left ventricle. The right coronary artery supplies the right atrium and ventricle and the left subdivides into the circumflex artery (supplying the left atrium and a portion of the left ventricle) and the anterior descending artery (supplying the remainder of the left ventricle and a small portion of the right ventricle). The deoxygenated blood is drained back into the right atrium via the coronary sinus.

1.9 Compare your labels to those on Fig. 1.8 (page 13).

1.10 60–100 beats per minute.

1.11 40–60 beats per minute.

1.12 20–40 beats per minute.

1.13 Blood enters the atria and raises the atrial pressure. When this exceeds the ventricular pressure, the AV valves open and most of the blood flows passively into the ventricles. The SA node fires causing atrial contraction and pushing out the remaining blood. Ventricular systole then occurs. When ventricular pressure exceeds atrial pressure, the AV valves close. When ventricular pressure exceeds aortic and pulmonary artery pressures, the semilunar valves open. Blood flows out of the ventricles into the pulmonary artery and aorta. Arterial pressure then exceeds ventricular pressure and the semilunar valves close. Ventricular diastole then occurs.

1.14 The vagus nerve supplies the heart. It is part of the parasympathetic nervous system, which slows the rate at which the SA node fires impulses, resulting in decreased rate and force of contraction. Sympathetic nerves increase the rate of impulse production from the SA node, to raise the rate and force of contraction.

1.15 A rise in blood pressure stimulates the baroreceptors to increase vagal tone (and lower heart rate). Adrenaline (epinephrine) and noradrenaline (norepinephrine) from the adrenal glands increase heart rate. Deep breathing stimulates the vagus nerve in the parasympathetic system and lowers heart rate. Hypoxia and hypercarbia decrease vagal tone so that sympathetic impulses become dominant and increase heart rate. A rise in body temperature affects the cardiac centre and increases heart rate. Thyroxine affects the SA node to raise the heart rate.

2: Principles of cardiac monitoring and the normal ECG

2.1 To pick up and display the electrical signals generated by the heart of any patient at risk of developing cardiac arrhythmias.

2.2 No, only the electrical activity.

2.3 Continuous cardiac monitoring (used to gain information about the patient's heart rate and rhythm); 12-lead ECG (used for precise diagnosis of cardiac problems); and defibrillator paddles (used in emergency situations only).

2.4 The red wire (positive lead) goes on the right shoulder; the yellow wire (negative lead) goes on the left shoulder; the green/black wire (ground lead) goes at the apex.

2.5 Lead II.

2.6 There is less interference.

2.7 Each very small square is 0.04 of a second.

2.8 Each small square is 0.20 of a second.

2.9 Each large square is 1 second.

2.10 The main ones relate to patient safety and accuracy of readings. The skin must be clean and dry. Lead II is used unless advised otherwise. Electrodes must be attached following local policy and kept moist and changed every 24 hours. The monitor must be easily seen and observed often for changes. The ECG trace must be clear and appropriate; check that it corresponds with the patient's apical rate. The monitor alarms must be set according to the patient's clinical condition. All changes must be documented and senior or medical staff informed of concerns.

2.11 The patient's breathing may affect the baseline. Make sure the electrodes aren't on the patient's lower ribs or that the patient isn't moving excessively. Replace electrodes that have been applied incorrectly.

2.12 Interference arises from electrical equipment (which should be kept as far away from the patient as possible) and electrodes that are not applied correctly (replace them). Artefacts are caused by shivering patients (keep them warm) or worn wires or cables (replace them).

2.13 This could be asystole (check the patient immediately and summon help and commence cardiopulmonary resuscitation if so). Some other causes include disconnected electrodes (replace them), too low a setting on the ECG gain (increase it), disconnected monitor leads (reconnect them), dried out gel on the electrodes (replace them), or worn out wires and cables (replace them).

2.14 The ECG complexes may be too small due to a weak signal (increase the gain), because of incorrectly placed electrodes (replace them) or because of worn wires or cables (replace them).

2.15 The gain may be set too high (reduce it), or the electrodes may not be applied correctly (replace them).

2.16 If the patient is OK, the alarm parameters are set too high or low, so they should be altered to an appropriate level. However, *never* turn off an alarm until you know why. And if in doubt – *shout*!

2.17 Do not use it because it could give the patient an electric shock. Get a new one!

2.18 Automaticity, excitability, conductivity and contractility.

2.19 Contractile and non-contractile.

2.20 Non-contractile cells.

2.21 Sodium (Na^+), potassium (K^+) and calcium (Ca^{++}).

2.22 Negative.

2.23 The cell membrane permeability changes and electrolytes move across it by diffusion or active transport. The inside of the cell becomes positively charged and it will therefore contract. The change in electrical potential of the myocardial cells as a result of the movement of electrolytes is known as the action potential.

2.24 Five.

2.25 Phase 0 to Phase 4. Phase 0 is rapid depolarisation; phase 1 is early repolarisation; phase 2 is the plateau phase; phase 3 is rapid repolarisation; and phase 4 is the resting phase.

2.26 During the *relative* refractory period a very strong electrical impulse can depolarise the cell early, but during the *absolute* refractory period not even a strong impulse will stimulate them.

2.27 Depolarisation.

2.28 Negative.

2.29 Each heart beat should be initiated by the SA node and made up of a P wave, a QRS complex and a T wave. The rhythm should be regular with rate around 72 b.p.m.

2.30 Atrial depolarisation, atrial repolarisation, ventricular depolarisation and ventricular repolarisation.

2.31 Atrial depolarisation.

2.32 Ventricular depolarisation.

2.33 Ventricular repolarisation.

2.34 Intervals contain waves but segments are the lines *between* the waves (where there is no electrical activity and the trace is isoelectric).

2.35 Compare your labels to those on Fig. 2.11 (page 32).

2.36 The time from the start of the P wave to the start of the QRS complex.

2.37 The time between the end of the P wave and the start of the QRS complex.

2.38 The time between the end of the S wave and the start of the T wave.

2.39 The time from the start of the Q wave to the end of the T wave.

2.40 Compare your labels with those on Fig. 2.13 (page 36).

2.41 Opposite.

2.42 Discuss your findings with your mentor.

3: Arrhythmia recognition

Information relating to Chapter 3 can be found in the answers for Chapter 5.

4: Arrhythmia interventions

4.1 Compare your table with Table 4.1 (pages 80–82).

4.2 Compare your table with Table 4.2 (pages 82–83).

4.3 By delivering a direct electrical current through the heart, which depolarises the myocardium and allows the sinoatrial node to resume its normal pacemaker function.

4.4 An automated external defibrillator – reliable, safe, computerised device that gives visual and voice prompts to rescuers and delivers defibrillatory shocks to patients in cardiac arrest.

4.5 They are attached to the defibrillator through an interface cable, rather than using paddles, so they reduce the risk of sparks and the operator does not have to lean over the patient.

4.6 The right (sternal electrode) goes below the clavicle to the right of the sternum. The apical paddle goes vertically in the mid-axillary line, level with the position of the V6 ECG electrode.

4.7 8 kg.

4.8 150–360 Joules.

4.9 Poorly applied paddles may cause a fire in an oxygen-rich environment so turn off oxygen supplementation or remove oxygen masks and nasal cannulae and move them at least one metre away before delivering a shock. Transdermal drug patches (e.g. GTN patches) may explode so remove them before delivering a shock. Sparking can occur, so use self-adhesive defibrillator pads rather than paddles where possible.

4.10 Cardioversion is carried out the same way as defibrillation but the DC shock is delivered in synchrony with the peak of the R wave. The defibrillator has a 'synchronise' switch which is used for cardioversion. The patient, if conscious, will usually require sedation with cardioversion. The intensity of the shock is usually less with cardioversion than with defibrillation.

4.11 The pacemaker device generates an electrical impulse which is transmitted through the heart causing depolarisation and muscular contraction.

4.12 In emergency and acute situations, until the arrhythmia has resolved, or until a permanent pacemaker can be fitted.

4.13 In emergency situations. One external electrode is applied to the anterior wall of the patient's chest, and another is applied to the patient's back. Electrical impulses pass through the skin to the myocardium.

4.14 In emergency situations. A pacing wire is passed into the right atrium or ventricle via the internal jugular or subclavian vein and attached to a pulse generator. Electrical impulses pass through the wire and stimulate the myocardium, causing it to depolarise and contract.

4.15 A pacing spike is visible on the ECG.

5: Putting it all together

5.1 Atrial fibrillation.

5.2 If the patient is unstable and the arrhythmia has been present for less than 48 hours, the treatment of choice is electrical cardioversion. If the ventricular rate is very rapid, carotid sinus massage may be useful for slowing the heart rate. If cardioversion does not convert the heart back to sinus rhythm, or if AF is persistent, pharmacologic conversion may be achieved with an intravenous antiarrhythmic agent, such as a class 1c drug like flecainide or propafenone – if there is no structural heart disease. If there is structural heart disease, use amiodarone. Also give anticoagulation because when the atria are fibrillating they do not empty correctly so there is an increased chance of clot formation.

5.3 This is not an arrhythmia. The gain is set too low so the ECG complexes are too small. The weak signal gives a false low reading.

5.4 Increase the gain and observe the trace. It is also possible that the electrodes are not applied correctly or the monitor wires or cables are worn so you should replace them or the monitor.

5.5 Multifocal ventricular extrasystoles (VEs).

5.6 If the VEs are infrequent and the patient is asymptomatic, no treatment is necessary. Frequent VEs and those causing symptoms of reduced cardiac output will require treatment and this will depend on the cause of the problem. For hypoxia, administer oxygen or increase oxygen concentration. For acidosis, correct the acidosis. For hypokalaemia, hypocalcaemia or hypomagnesaemia provide intravenous supplementation. Frequent or dangerous VEs will require antiarrhythmic drugs. Intravenous amiodarone and beta-blockers and calcium-channel blockers can be used.

5.7 Mobitz type I second-degree heart block (Wenckebach phenomenon).

5.8 If the patient is asymptomatic, the heart block is usually transient and does not require treatment. However, delayed conduction signifies a problem in the conducting system, so this should be monitored. The underlying cause should be treated because a Mobitz type I block can progress to more serious forms of heart block. For prolonged rhythm causing a reduction in cardiac output, atropine or a temporary pacing wire may be needed.

5.9 Sinus bradycardia.

5.10 If the patient is asymptomatic, no treatment is necessary for sinus bradycardia. A heart rate of less than 60 b.p.m. may result in collapse or symptoms of inadequate perfusion. If there is a sudden bradycardia, the adult bradycardia algorithm should be used. Do an ABC assessment and ensure the patient's airway is clear, and give oxygen and respiratory assistance if required. Use transcutaneous or transvenous pacing, using drugs like atropine or inotropic agents to support the patient's circulation prior to pacing.

5.11 Polymorphic ventricular tachycardia (VT).

5.12 Management depends on the symptoms. Pulseless patients are treated as for ventricular fibrillation, using cardiopulmonary resuscitation and defibrillation following the UK Resuscitation Council's algorithm. If the pulse is present but the patient is unstable, use DC synchronised cardioversion immediately. Treat stable patients with amiodarone and correct the cause. If amiodarone doesn't work, perform DC synchronised cardioversion.

5.13 Atrial tachycardia.

5.14 If the arrhythmia is transient and the patient is asymptomatic, no treatment is necessary but he or she should be observed. Any underlying cause should be treated. A sustained tachycardia, even in an asymptomatic patient, should be treated. Depending on how unstable the patient is, give amiodarone or use electrical cardioversion. Carotid sinus massage can sometimes successfully slow the heart rate in the first instance.

5.15 Unifocal ventricular extrasystoles (VEs).

5.16 If they are infrequent and the patient is asymptomatic no treatment is needed. Frequent VEs and those causing symptoms of reduced cardiac output, will have to be treated. For patients with hypoxia, give oxygen or increase oxygen concentration. For patients with acidosis, correct the acidosis. For patients with low potassium, calcium or magnesium give intravenous supplements. For frequent and/or dangerous VEs, give antiarrhythmic drugs (intravenous amiodarone, beta-blockers and/or calcium-channel blockers).

5.17 Bigeminy.

5.18 If runs of bigeminy are infrequent and the patient is asymptomatic, no treatment is necessary. Frequent runs of bigeminy and those that produce symptoms of reduced cardiac output require to be treated, again depending on the cause. Administer or increase oxygen; correct any acidosis; supplement any ion deficiencies; or instigate antiarrhythmic therapy

5.19 Monomorphic ventricular tachycardia (VT).

5.20 This depends on the symptoms. If the patient is pulseless, treat as for ventricular fibrillation (defibrillation and cardiopulmonary resuscitation). If a pulse is present but the patient is unstable, perform DC synchronised cardioversion. Stable patients can be given amiodarone and if this fails, DC synchronised cardioversion must be performed.

5.21 R-on-T phenomenon.

5.22 If it is caused by hypoxia, oxygen administration is required or increased oxygen concentration. Any acidosis must be corrected and supplements given to correct low levels of potassium, calcium or magnesium. Because it is potentially dangerous, intravenous amiodarone should be given. Beta-blockers and calcium-channel blockers may also be used.

5.23 Atrial flutter.

5.24 If the patient is unstable, synchronous DC cardioversion is the usual initial treatment. An antiarrhythmic agent, beta-blocker or calcium-channel blocker may be used if symptoms are less severe. If the heart rate is high, it may be necessary to terminate the arrhythmia by inserting a temporary pacing wire.

5.25 Coarse ventricular fibrillation (VF).

5.26 If VF is suspected, immediately check the patient. Remember VF can be mimicked by external electrical interference. If the patient is unresponsive, instigate defibrillation immediately following the UK Resuscitation Council's algorithm, as the patient is in cardiac arrest. A single precordial thump may be given when cardiac arrest is confirmed after a sudden collapse (if no defibrillator is available). Cardiopulmonary resuscitation must be initiated if defibrillation is delayed for any reason to ensure oxygen delivery. Administer intravenous epinephrine if defibrillation does not immediately restore sinus rhythm.

5.27 Premature atrial contractions (PACs).

5.28 If the patient has no cardiac disease and is asymptomatic, treatment is rarely necessary. If the PACs are caused by a removable cause (caffeine, alcohol or other such irritants) advise the patient to reduce intake. Patients with an underlying disease and symptoms from the PACs, should be given a drug like digoxin to increase the atrial refractory period.

5.29 This is not an arrhythmia but a wandering baseline.

5.30 This may be caused by the patient's breathing, so make sure the electrodes are not on the patient's lower ribs. If the patient is moving excessively, encourage him or her to remain calm and still. Replace any electrodes that are not applied correctly.

5.31 Sinus tachycardia.

5.32 If there is no underlying cause, the tachycardia is transient and the patient is asymptomatic, then no treatment is necessary – just observe the patient. Sustained sinus tachycardia, even in asymptomatic patients, should be treated. If the cause is haemorrhage or hypovolaemia, stop the bleeding and replace fluid. Other causes may be treated with beta-blockers or calcium-channel blockers. Critically ill patients may require circulatory support from inotropic agents that increase cardiac contractility.

5.33 This is not an arrhythmia. It is caused by artefact/electrical interference.

5.34 Artefact may be caused by shivering, so keep the patient warm. Electrical equipment near the patient may cause problems so it should be moved as far from the patient as possible. The electrodes may not be applied correctly or the monitor wires or cables may be worn, so they must be replaced.

5.35 Fine ventricular fibrillation (VF).

5.36 VF can be mimicked by external electrical interference, but in suspected VF you should immediately check the patient. If he or she is unresponsive, start defibrillation immediately (the patient is in cardiac arrest). If there is doubt about whether the rhythm is asystole or fine VF, do not attempt defibrillation; instead, continue chest compression and ventilation. Consider giving a single precordial thump when cardiac arrest is confirmed rapidly after a witnessed and monitored sudden collapse, and a defibrillator is not immediately available. Initiate cardiopulmonary resuscitation if defibrillation is delayed to maintain oxygen delivery. Administer intravenous epinephrine if defibrillation does not immediately revert to sinus rhythm.

5.37 This is not an arrhythmia. The gain is set too high giving a false high reading.

5.38 Reduce the gain and observe the trace. Also check whether the electrodes have been applied correctly.

5.39 Sinus arrhythmia.

5.40 Unless the patient is symptomatic, this is no cause for concern and requires no treatment. If there is an underlying cause, it should be monitored and dealt with.

5.41 Sinus rhythm.

5.42 This is the normal rhythm of the heart and therefore it requires no treatment. However, critically ill patients should still be monitored and observed closely, as changes in rhythm can occur suddenly.

5.43 Asystole.

5.44 If asystole is suspected, check the patient *immediately*. It can be mimicked by something as simple as electrode detachment. Ensure that fine ventricular fibrillation is excluded by turning up the gain on the monitor. If the patient is pulseless and unresponsive, cardiopulmonary resuscitation must be instigated immediately together with a single dose of intravenous atropine and repeated doses of epinephrine (adrenaline) following the UK Resuscitation Council's algorithm.

5.45 Third-degree heart block.

5.46 In a critically ill patient, this arrhythmia will usually drastically reduce cardiac output and is a medical emergency. It requires immediate drug therapy, aimed at improving the ventricular rate. Atropine is usually given and inotropic agents may be required to support the patient's circulation. The insertion of a temporary pacing wire is often necessary until the cause of the block has been resolved. If the block is permanent, a permanent pacemaker will subsequently be needed.

5.47 Trigeminy.

5.48 If runs of trigeminy are infrequent and the patient is asymptomatic, no treatment is necessary. However, if they are frequent and/or produce symptoms of reduced cardiac output, treatment will need to be instigated. The treatment depends upon the cause of the problem. For example, if caused by hypoxia, oxygen administration is required or increase oxygen concentration; if caused by acidosis, correct the acidosis. Ventricular extrasystoles may be caused by hypokalaemia (low potassium), hypocalcaemia (low calcium) or hypomagnesaemia (low magnesium), and therefore intravenous supplementation will be required. If the runs of trigeminy are frequent and/or dangerous, antiarrhythmic drugs may be required. Intravenous amiodarone is used for the acute treatment of trigeminy. Beta-blockers and calcium-channel blockers may also be used.

5.49 Junctional escape rhythm.

5.50 If the patient is asymptomatic, generally this rhythm is not treated, but – if necessary – the underlying cause is. In patients with complete heart block, or symptomatic sick sinus syndrome, a permanent pacemaker may be needed. An anticholinergic drug such as atropine may be required if symptomatic bradycardia is present.

5.51 First-degree heart block.

5.52 If the patient is asymptomatic, this heart block is not treated. However, a delay in conduction means there is a problem in the conducting system and therefore the patient should be monitored. The underlying cause should be treated if necessary because first-degree block can progress to more serious forms of heart block.

5.53 Mobitz type II second-degree heart block.

5.54 Transcutaneous pacing or a temporary transvenous pacing wire is indicated for all patients with Mobitz type II blocks, including asymptomatic patients, because patients with this kind of block usually progress to complete heart block. An anticholinergic, such as atropine, may also be required.

5.55 Discuss the six samples you collected and analysed with your mentor.

5.56 Discuss the six samples you collected and analysed with your mentor.

References

Adgey, A.A.J. (2005). *The role of biphasic shocks for transthoracic cardioversion of atrial fibrillation*. Available at: http://cogprints.org/4595/1/adgey.htm (last accessed January 2010).

Beinart, S.C., Rosero, S., Zareba, W. and Huang, D. (2006). *Junctional rhythm: treatment and medication*. Available at: http://emedicine.medscape.com/article/155146-treatment (last accessed January 2010).

British Medical Association and Royal Pharmaceutical Society of Great Britain (2009). *British National Formulary, No. 57*. London: BMA/RPSGB. Available at: http://www.bnf.org (last accessed January 2010)

Bruck, L., Donofrio, J., Munden, J. and Thompson, G. (eds) (2005). *Anatomy and Physiology made Incredibly Easy*, 2nd edn. London: Lippincott, Williams and Wilkins.

Cowley, M. (2006). *Electrodes, leads and wires: A practical guide to ECG monitoring and recording*. Available at: http://www.mikecowley.co.uk/leads.htm (last accessed January 2010).

Davis, D. (2005). *12-Lead ECG Interpretation*, 4th edn. London: Lippincott, Williams and Wilkins.

Docherty, B. and Douglas, M. (2003). Cardiac care 3: ECG interpretation. Ventricular arrhythmias. *Professional Nurse* **18**(8), 459–61.

Foxall, F. (2009). *Haemodynamic Monitoring and Manipulation*. Cumbria: M&K Publishing.

Gonce-Morton, P., Fontaine, D.K., Hudak, C.M. and Gallo, B.M. (2005). *Critical Care Nursing: A Holistic Approach*, 8th edn. London: Lippincott, Williams and Wilkins.

Hand, H. (2002). Common cardiac arrhythmias. *Emergency Nurse* **10**(3), 29–38.

Haworth, K., Mayer, B.H., Mundon, J., Munson, C., Schaeffer, L. and Wittig, P. (eds) (2004). *Critical Care Nursing Made Incredibly Easy*. London: Lippincott, Williams and Wilkins.

Jaeger, F.J. (2008). *Cardiac arrhythmias*. Available at: http://www.clevelandclinicmeded.com/medicalpubs/diseasemanagement/cardiology/cardiac-arrhythmias/ (last accessed January 2010).

Jansen, J.R.C. (2002). An adequate strategy for the thermodilution technique in patients during mechanical ventilation. *Intensive Care Medicine* 6, 422.

Janson-Cohen, B. (2005). *Memmler's The Human Body in Health and Disease*, 10th edn. London: Lippincott, Williams and Wilkins.

Jevon, P. and Ewens, B. (eds) (2007). *Monitoring the Critically Ill Patient*, 2nd edn. Oxford: Blackwell Science.

Lazar, J. and Clark, A.D. (2007). *Atrial fibrillation: Treatment and medication*. Available at: http://emedicine.medscape.com/article/757370–treatment (last accessed January 2010).

Lazar, J. and Parwani, V. (2006). *Atrial flutter: Treatment and medication*. Available at: http://emedicine.medscape.com/article/757549-treatment (last accessed January 2010).

Levine, J., Munden, J. and Thompson, G. (2008). *ECG Interpretation Made Incredibly Easy*, 4th edn. London: Lippincott, Williams and Wilkins.

Levine, M.D. and Brown, D.F.M. (2006). *Heart block, second degree: Treatment and medication*. Available at: http://emedicine.medscape.com/article/758383-treatment (last accessed January 2010).

Marieb, E.N. (2006). *Essentials of Human Anatomy and Physiology*, 8th edn. London: Pearson.

Marini, J.J. and Wheeler, A.P. (2006). *Critical Care Medicine*, 3rd edn. London: Lippincott, Williams and Wilkins.

Martini, F.H. (2006). *Fundamentals of Anatomy and Physiology*, 7th edn. London: Pearson.

Martini, F.H. and Bartholomew, E.F. (2007). *Essentials of Anatomy and Physiology*, 4th edn. London: Pearson Education.

Mattson-Porth, C. (2005). *Pathophysiology: Concepts of Altered Health States*, 7th edn. London: Lippincott, Williams and Wilkins.

National Institute for Health and Clinical Excellence (2006). *CG36 NICE Guideline: Atrial fibrillation*. Available at: http://guidance.nice.org.uk/CG36/NiceGuidance/doc/English (last accessed January 2010).

Resuscitation Council UK (2009). *Resuscitation Guidelines 2005*. Available at: http://www.resus.org.uk (last accessed January 2010).

Vaughan-Williams E.M. (1970). Classification of anti-arrhythmic drugs. In: E. Sandfte, E. Flensted-Jensen, K.H. Olesen (eds) *Symposium on Cardiac Arrhythmias*. Sweden, AB ASTRA, Södertälje.

Viney, C. (1999) *Nursing the Critically Ill*. London: Bailliere Tindall.

Index